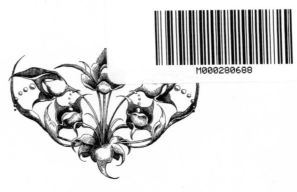

IN PRAISE OF

Mama's Home Remedies

"The suggestions in this volume bring fruitful advice and invaluable worth. Most people have forgotten that the simple things are at the center of soulful nurturing and this health publication is an exemplary model of such authentic knowledge. This book offers us an outline of happiness and health. Everyone will benefit from these jewels of understanding and I am sure that you will be as rewarded as I was after embracing many of these natural prescriptions."

—*Anna Maria Clement, PhD, NMD, codirector and chief health administrator of Hippocrates Health Institute*

"I thoroughly enjoyed reading "Dialogue with the Trees of Strength and Everlasting Life" in Mama's Home Remedies. *Svetlana Konnikova fills this delightful essay on the importance of trees in our lives with fascinating legends, appealing real-life personal and family stories, poetry, home remedies, interesting nature facts, and motivating aphorisms. She even includes a chart of the Trees of Life; mine is the walnut, the tree of passion and power. Her descriptions of scenery paint colorful pictures that make me want to go to the places she portrays. I am proud that she quotes from my grandfather Joyce Kilmer's poem, "Trees." I hope that her work will help to instill a deeper reverence for the environment in readers everywhere."*

—*Miriam A. Kilmer, artist and granddaughter of poet Joyce Kilmer, author of "Trees"*

Mama's
Home Remedies

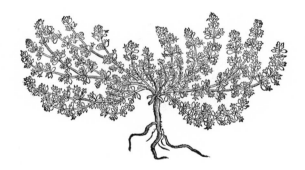

Never does nature say one thing and wisdom another.

— *Juvenal (A.D. 50-130), Roman Writer*

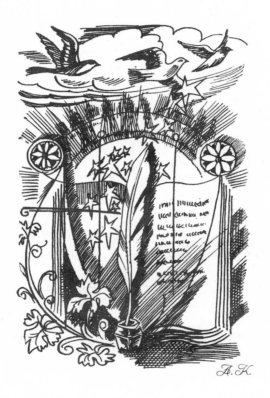

An expert is a man who has made all the mistakes which can be made in a very narrow field.

—Niels Bohr (1885–1962), Danish physicist and Nobel Laureate

Mama's Home Remedies

*Discover Time-Tested Secrets of Good Health
and the Pleasures of Natural Living*

Svetlana Konnikova, MA, AN

Foreword by Anna Maria Clement, PhD, NMD

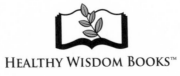

HEALTHY WISDOM BOOKS™

An Imprint of AURORA PUBLISHERS

HEALTHY WISDOM BOOKS™

PUBLISHED BY AURORA PUBLISHERS, INC.

$\mathcal{M}ama's$ Home Remedies

Copyright © 2008 by Svetlana Konnikova. All rights reserved.
Cover photograph Copyright © Richard T. Nowitz /SuperStock, Inc.

Illustrations by Alexander Khmelnitsky and Anatoli Smishliaev.
Used by permission.

Konnikova, Svetlana

Mama's Home Remedies/ Svetlana Konnikova

p.cm
Includes Index

Hardcover
ISBN: 978-0-9791758-1-7
LCCN: 2007906435

Paperback
ISBN: 978-0-9791758-2-4
LCCN: 2007932536

1. Health. 2. Natural Healing. 3. Herbs, Plants. 4. Mind, Body, Spirit.
5. Cookery. 1. Title.

Available wherever books are sold, or order from
Independent Publishers Group:
Call toll-free: 800-888-4741
Fax: 312-337-5985
Email: orders@ipgbook.com

Visit our website at www.aurorapublishers.com

Printed in the United States of America
Published January 2008
First edition
10 9 8 7 6 5 4 3 2

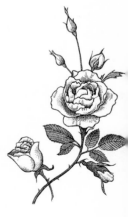

CONTENTS

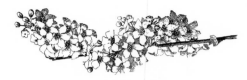

IMPORTANT NOTICE

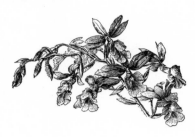

The information and recommendations in this book have been practically tested and proven by many people. However, the information contained herein is to be used as a reference source only. The author of this book is not a physician and the procedures, ideas, and suggestions in this book are not intended as a substitute for the medical advice of a trained health professional. Some herbs and plants used as remedies or food, internally or externally, can cause allergic reactions in some individuals. These methods should not be used for long-term problems and serious illness. Consult your doctor or qualified health-care practitioner before adapting the suggestions in this book. Always seek the advice of your physician about any condition that may require diagnosis or medical treatment.

The statements made by the author regarding certain products and services represent the views of the author alone, and do not constitute a recommendation or endorsement of any product or service by the publisher. The author and publisher disclaim any liability arising directly or indirectly from the use of the book. Neither the author nor the publisher can be held responsible for claims arising from the inappropriate use of any remedy in this book or from the mistaken identity of any herbs or other components of the recipes herein.

PREFACE

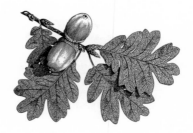

ama's Home Remedies is an easy-to-read, learn-and-do practical guide written for people unfamiliar with the basics of common herbal remedies but who wish to derive benefits from the medicinal properties of herbs. These herbs have been healing peoples of the world—Sumerians and Babylonians six thousand years before the Common Era; Scythians (second and third centuries B.C.E.), the first and oldest tribes of ancient Greece and Russia; and Egyptians four thousand years ago.

This book is written for everybody who has a desire to improve his or her health naturally. Hundreds of natural treatments, small real-life anecdotes, and inspirational notes are garnered from the personal observations, experience, and life philosophy of several generations of women in one family and their friends, passed down through centuries.

The therapeutic properties of more than 100 medicinal herbs, plants, and trees are examined herein along with the true, lyrical and romantic memoirs of a family who for many years supported each other. Life experience is paralleled with ancient mythology and Grandma's folk tales, fairy tales and legends.

FOREWORD

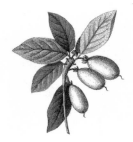

Svetlana Konnikova has penned an important book using the wisdom of the ages for the age in which we live. Her time-tested, natural remedies were born out of necessity in generations past when the pharmaceutical approach was not available. This hearty group was fortunate to live off of the earth, from the earth and wholly healthfully. Most often, it was our grandmothers and mothers who nursed us back from sickness and on rare occasions they may have seen the village or town's doctor who also used herbs, food and love as a remedy. Each ethnic culture developed their own natural pharmacy determined by their unique environment, long history and personal needs. Svetlana's northern European offerings are sophisticated since these hearty people who lived in severe conditions manifested an equally strong system of earth's healthcare.

The suggestions in this volume bring fruitful advice and invaluable worth. It is impressive to note the thoughtfulness and maternal care that was taken in weaving this guide together. As a native European who has worked in complimentary healthcare in North America for decades, I can confirm the value of this priceless counsel. Most people have forgotten that the simple things are at the center of soulful nurturing and this health publication is an exemplary model of such authentic knowledge. As days pass, modern people are rushing toward the edge of a precipice. It is abundantly clear to any thinking person that we must halt this self-destructive pattern and once again come to our senses. Each of us must take personal responsibility for all aspects of our lives; most importantly, our physical, emotional, mental and spiritual health.

We can change the course of our future, either making it a pathway of fulfillment and abundant joy or an excruciating voyage through the misery of irresponsibility. In your hands, you hold an important key to the place where all of us wish to reside. This special space is free from suffering and filled with health. Do not allow commercial interests to rob you of inherent strength by selling you inferior and destructive products and ideas. Help yourself by increasing your know-how and succeeding with your conquest. This accumulating character-building continuum gives you the wherewithal to engage wholeness. When you have achieved this crucial plateau, the insight and tools will be available so that you can build the necessary health that is required to live a full and successful life. Ms. Konnikova should be congratulated for her laborious efforts to offer us an outline to happiness and health. Everyone will benefit from these jewels of understanding and I am sure that you will be as rewarded as I was after embracing many of these natural prescriptions.

Anna Maria Clement, PhD, NMD
Codirector and Chief Health Administrator
of Hippocrates Health Institute, West Palm Beach, Florida

INTRODUCTION

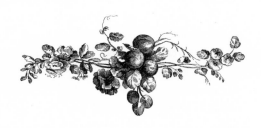

*If I were to name the three most precious resources of life,
I should say books, friends, and nature. Nature we have always
with us, an inexhaustible storehouse of that which moves the heart,
appeals to the mind, and fires the imagination—health to the body,
a stimulus to the intellect, and joy to the soul.*

—John Burroughs (1837–1921), American writer and naturalist

My interest in herbs and nature began long ago. I remember my first impression: a bunch of small chamomile flowers in a crystal vase standing on a side table near my bed. They held a delicate aroma that I memorized forever. I feel that it blends perfectly with my body chemistry.

Chamomile was the first of Nature's greetings to me from the unknown, miraculous world outside. I grew up in a home filled with dried herbs, potted plants, and fragrant sachets everywhere to keep the air fresh with an energizing scent. Our kitchen was filled with numerous packets and glass jars of mixed herbs, *nastoykas* (infusions), juices, teas, and elixirs.

Beginning with my great-great-grandmother, several generations of women in our family were fascinated with herbs and everything that Nature could provide us. Grandma planted herbs, flowers, and trees in her gardens and used them as natural healers in the preparation of homemade green medicines; as cosmetics; and in cooking delicious vegetable meals, preserves, and jams.

All the women in our family, except my mother, were homemakers, but they learned how to use a green pharmacy. They acquired a broad range of knowledge of plants and used it to prevent and heal various ailments in their family members.

Generation after generation accepted the importance of herbs in healing naturally, in eating healthy foods, and in keeping themselves at their best. They also explored the incredible world of Nature in another part of our house. Our family library contained hundreds of books. My grandmother and grandfather, and then my parents, created an exciting atmosphere there where my aunts and uncles, cousins, good friends, and neighbors were welcomed to tea parties and "green" dinners, where candlelight and stimulating conversations abounded.

My sister and I grew up without extensive use of antibiotics and other drugs. Instead we were surrounded with great books, good friends, a beautiful natural environment, Grandma's fairy tales, and her green-blue garden. We also had Grandpa's wisdom and his vineyards with ripe grapes, Papa's home library with hundreds of great books and lessons on how to reach your dreams, and Mama's motivational discussions on self-esteem and treatment with her homemade healing remedies.

I read many medical books from Mama's library and she shared with me her knowledge. She often told me, "You are a doctor by nature. It is a gift from God. You understand and feel the nature of disease. Why won't you continue to study medicine?"

"Mama, my first love is journalism," I would tell her.

Although I felt a strong desire to devote my life to becoming a doctor, I dreamed also of being a journalist. I was torn between the two paths and had such a difficult time making one "right" choice that I chose a "gold middle."

I became a writer and a broadcast journalist, an educator, and the family "doctor" for my husband and two sons. I feel comfortable sharing the knowledge I've garnered from Grandma and Mama's wisdom combined with my own research and formal education, including the study of natural remedies from fifteenth-century herbal books through current advances.

Many of the hundreds of Mama's recipes have been used widely in Russia and Europe for centuries. I am happy now to share with you my knowledge and show you how you can treat illnesses in a wise way without polluting your body with an endless flow of chemicals.

Svetlana Konnikova

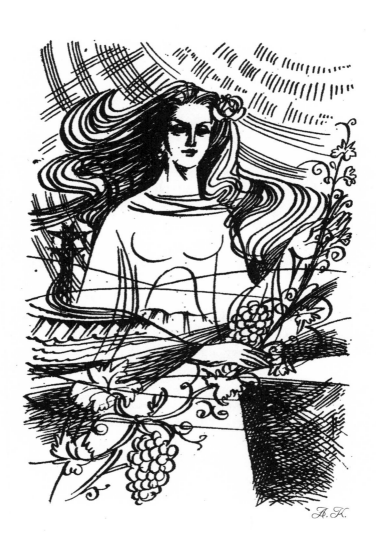

A Fine Mood

Who was silent by the window?
Fog quarreled with rain
and it was a long, long evening…
about something far away, unearthly,
about something close and kindred.
The weeping candles burn down.
And what is there to cry about?
All in all, we are in fact alive,
but sometimes toward evening
suddenly we feel sorry for ourselves.
It's always toward evening
and we sit down at the grand piano,
lift a veil from the keyboard,
and bring the candles back to life.
These candles weep for the people –
now softly, now intense,
unable to quench their tears
in time.
It's very important for me
that we have no fear of fire,
that the candles cry for the people,
burn down and, soundless, melt away.
Tomorrow daylight comes again,
and we'll hear a tune again,
like Mama's song.
And a musician will be playing
to make the people glad again.
And like a song it comes back to you
that fine mood.

S. K.

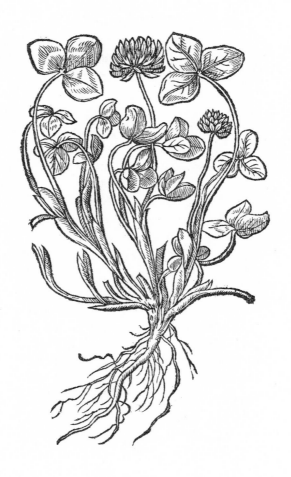

Chapter 1

Rose Hips Tea Party

To live we need sun, freedom and a small flower.

—*Hans Christian Andersen (1805-1875), Danish writer*

Tea parties were a Friday tradition and always a perfect get-together at our home. The "girls" would meet as usual in our garden. They were my mother's girlfriends, medical professionals, doctors, and nurses. They worked together many years and shared one love, an obsession with their medical profession.

During these years they accumulated a rich experience in healing people from different diseases. They were a team of courageous and noble people whom I observed and from whom I learned. I listened to their long conversations about natural healing and alternative medicine and their humorous stories with unabated attention. I was 12 when I began to keep a journal in which I wrote my observations and collected valuable information that I gleaned from Mama and her friends.

They told me that whenever they began to work with any patient, they would recite to them this ancient parable:

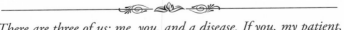

There are three of us: me, you, and a disease. If you, my patient, will be on the side of illness, I will not overcome you as a doctor. If you will be on my side, together we will conquer your illness.

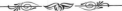

Mama's and her friends' practice was evidence that this psychological approach worked. It was motivation for the people to fight their illnesses. It was a clear direction to health and life. The "girls" gathered these miraculous remedies from centuries of wisdom and expertise including their own mothers, grandmothers, and Mother Nature. They combined the natural method of physical therapy with electro-physiology. They prescribed well-known antibiotics and other drugs, but their first attempt to heal a patient was always with the sole use of herbal remedies.

Tea was considered to be an essential part of *l' art de vivre*. They sat down to tea many times—the same party around the same table on our patio, overlooking Grandma's multicolored garden with an array of flowers that greeted them with sweet and pungent aromas while the strains of Tchaikovsky's "Waltz of the Flowers" filled the air.

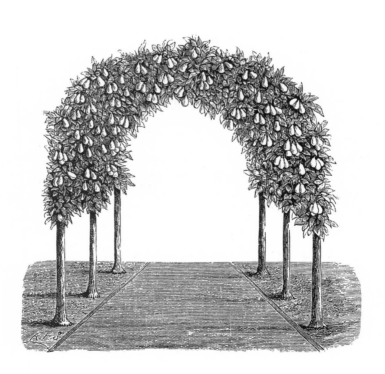

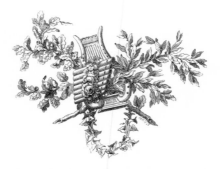

To live happily is an inward power of the soul.

—*Marcus Aurelius (A.D. 161-180), Roman emperor*

Mama's Philosophy for Your Motivation

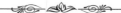

- Life is a beautiful gift given to all of us. We should use it properly.

- Be kind and try to do something good for somebody right now. Don't delay because we will not pass the same way again.

- Be an attentive listener and motivator if family members or your friends share their ultimate secrets, goals, and dreams with you. Never put them down. The consequences can be unpredictable.

- Be positive and constructive. Be straightforward and encouraging. As a result, something great can come out of it.

- Look at the sunny side of everything in your life and be optimistic. Your optimism will become reality.

- Make your life an example of health, happiness, and prosperity. This will give you an opportunity to become a knowledgeable advisor and expert.

- Be generous. Share your rich experience with those who would like to take advantage of it.

- Be really responsible for your life and follow your heart.

- Our life is a gift twice: once for ourselves and once for others.

- Our life is a mirror in which we can see good and bad. Our health is a shield—physical and mental. Our physical health has an influence on our spiritual life, but our spiritual power gives us the discipline required to maintain our health.

- Our health and our well-being rest in our hands.

- Think only of the best and build your long and happy life, based on the laws of Nature.

- Chase your goals and perform good deeds.

- Be strong and have the guts to say "No" when you feel that something is not right. The world will not change to suit your preferences.

- Be a very good sport to your family and friends. Love, inspire, amuse, and believe in them. It is mutual. You'll get the same treatment back.

- Consider every day as a small life and each day as full and perfect.

- Be confident that nothing can disturb your peace of mind. Be strong against fear.

- Be noble and mighty against jealousy and anger.

- Help others in need of your help, and just do it!

- To live a long, healthy, and happy life is an art—*l' art de vivre*.

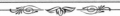

Chapter 2

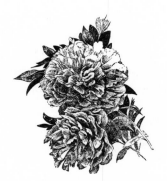

"Even the Badger Knows . . ."

Nature is to be found in her entirety nowhere more than in her smallest creatures.

—*Pliny the Elder (A.D. 23-79), Roman scholar*

FACTS:

More than one-third of U.S. citizens use natural medicine today. The government has suggested that more and more people became interested in herbs, meditation, yoga, and other forms of alternative medicine because they don't see positive results very often with conventional care.

One of the largest U.S. studies conducted on alternative medicine found that over ⅓ of American adults practiced some type of alternative medicine in 2002. The report was based on information from 31,044 interviews with adults age 18 or older.

Researchers believe that results of the study point to the fact that more people are using alternative medicine and an increasing number of people have turned to natural products like herbs, fruits, vegetables, or enzymes to help treat chronic or recurring pain.

Experts suggest that people should not neglect conventional medicine in those cases where it has been proven to help certain conditions. They also recommend consulting a doctor before practicing alternative medicine. Experts express concern about the number of people turning to alternative medicine because they felt they were no longer able to pay the costs of conventional care. Experts also caution people to be careful before they use a natural product and not assume that it is automatically safe to consume only because it is natural. The study cited an example that 6.6 percent of people in the study used the supplement kava kava, which has been linked to liver disease.

The study found that 62 percent of the participants used some form of complimentary or alternative medicine over the past year for a specific medical condition:

- 43 percent prayed for their own health
- 24 percent were prayed for by others
- 19 percent used herbs, other natural and botanical products, and enzymes
- 12 percent practiced deep breathing exercises
- 10 percent participated in group prayer for their own health
- 8 percent used meditation
- 8 percent sought chiropractic care
- 5 percent practiced yoga
- 5 percent used massage
- 4 percent implemented diet-based therapies

Research showed that there was a higher tendency for women to use complementary and alternative medicine than men. Twenty-eight percent of the participants felt that conventional treatment would not help them.[1]

I can still hear Mama's refrain whenever she administered one of her wonderful, healing herbs to me or to my sister. "Even the badger knows that Mother Nature is the best healer," she would say with a knowing smile. Our friends and family used this phrase frequently. It was popular among "the girls," Mama's friends, and, in turn, their children grew fond of it and used it as well. Thus, the saying along with an understanding of the use of healing herbs became like a fine, gold chain connecting friends and family together in pursuit of natural, herbal remedies for prevention of and the treatment of illnesses.

We first encountered the phrase in a lyrical story, "The Badger's Nose," written by the Russian writer Konstantin Paustovsky in 1935. I can hardly believe that this brilliant writer wrote this piece during Stalin's rule, a period filled with fear and repression. Fortunately he was not punished and sent to Stalin's prison camps as were many other people who chose to express, rather than repress, their views. Perhaps it lies in the fact that Paustovsky focused his writings on beautiful, short stories about Nature, animals, trees, and his profound love for our planet.

His story takes us back to our natural roots and explains how the bold and wise badger used his instincts to survive by foraging for just the right "medicine" from Nature's green pharmacy.

I first heard Mama's version of this story when I was a child. When I had my own children, I too adapted the story to my own words, so I told them my version and they understood what it means to be in harmony with Nature and all she provides. They admired how the small and clever badger successfully treated and healed his wounds by using natural resources. It became my children's favorite and they requested it time and again. Each time the story is told by someone new, the words are bound to change, but the moral remains crystal clear. *Trust in Nature to be healed.*

You will be able to read my variation of Paustovsky's classic story of delicate psychological insight that speaks of a small animal that we, depending on where we live, can sometimes see in our own backyards, in the forthcoming book, *The Badger's Nose.*

The badger knows that Mother Nature is the best healer. Thus, if you love Nature, you can easily explore her green pharmacy. Look in your kitchen cupboard for yellow onion, garlic, cabbage, or ginger.

- Rub the highly antiseptic cloves of garlic (peeled and cut open) on acne pustules and other infected pimples.
- Crush garlic and apply to stubborn corns to draw them out. Fold a bandage into three layers with the garlic in between and roll over the finger or toe.
- Cut one slice of yellow onion and put it on insect stings—you'll get rapid relief.
- Lie down and apply washed fresh cabbage leaves as a plaster to the forehead and temples for 15 minutes to soothe a burn or bruise or to relieve headaches.

✍ Chew a piece of crystallized ginger or eat ginger candy or cookies to prevent travel sickness such as nausea and vomiting during long journeys in a car or boat.

Go with your children to the national parks, forests, meadows, lakes, wetlands, and swamps. You will discover a whole new world there. Ask questions! Healthy curiosity brings its own rewards.

In a countryside emergency you can apply yarrow leaves to wounds and nosebleeds. Lie down for 15–20 minutes or wrap a bandage or cheesecloth around your wound. With nosebleeds you must lie down for 10–15 minutes at least. Do the same with crushed daisies and it will help you with bruises and sprains. Fresh leaves of shepherd's purse, Self-Heal, or wild geranium will stop bleeding. Use the same method with the bandage or cheesecloth or lie down until the bleeding stops.

It has been always a mystery how animals follow their instincts and recognize the healing properties of plants, especially those which can treat their wounds, burns, scratches, and bites of other stronger animals.

Guess what? They never had doctors or pills, like we do. However they also want to survive on the planet Earth, so Mother Nature gave all Earth's inhabitants her generous gifts—plants, herbs, trees, and flowers. She planted them everywhere—in gardens, forests, meadows, glades, fields, swamps, and marshes. She created the world's most amazing huge green hospital where remedies for health problems are 100 percent natural and grow right under your feet so people and animals can use them any time and heal themselves.

I don't know many people who have enough knowledge to take advantage of this free "hospital," but the animals know for sure what to do and how to take care of themselves. They know which "green medicines" are safe and which are poisonous. They have amazing instincts for survival, much better than people have. The explanation is quite simple: they are born and live in a wild environment and must rely on themselves.

From our story you will learn how the badger treated his nose, badly burned in boiling hot oil, with the mold from the decomposed stump of a pine tree.

We too have the ability to explore Nature's green pharmacy and learn how to be healthier and happier. Good luck to you on the road to explore a new you!

Natural medicine recognizes the healing properties of plants, minerals, and different stones. However, for centuries scientists and doctors ignored unusual treatments employed by so-called "ignorant" healers. These remedies include mold and spider's web or gossamer. Most doctors and scientists discounted them. In the meantime "women from the crowd" (midwives) treated inflammation with these natural antiseptics—just as our little hero, the badger, did.

What is this miraculous mold from the decomposed stump of a pine tree? You'll be disappointed if you expect to see something beautiful. This green mold looks very unattractive. It was called "an awful green mold or mud," even by some bright scientists. For years it was considered to be harmful and even infectious and useless and it was scorned by good doctors.

Many years ago a physician in Russia was shocked to see that his patient had used an awful green mold as a substitute for a medicinal ointment.

"Look, this is only one step away from gangrene!" he exclaimed indignantly.

But after inspecting the patient's wound, he had to admit that the wound had healed. The doctor was greatly surprised and said, "I don't get it! This is either mysticism or a smart witch did a great job."

He added. "You are really lucky, sir. Are you aware of that? Your body is perfectly healthy, and you have successfully overcome this pathogenic infection—even under the harmful influence of this green mud. You could have contracted a life-threatening blood poisoning or sepsis."

This sort of prejudice has prevailed for many years. An awful green mold or mud was scorned by doctors even long after Sir Alexander Fleming, a British bacteriologist, discovered the antibiotic qualities of the lysozyme in 1922 and the mold fungus penicillin in 1928. Lysozyme is an enzyme present in human body tissues and it is lethal to certain bacteria. This discovery at first prepared the way for antibiotics.

Later Fleming made a great discovery with penicillin and scientifically proved its valuable antibiotic qualities. Then penicillin was developed as a therapeutic drug by Lord Howard Walter Florey and Sir Ernst Boris Chain. All three scientists received the 1945 Nobel Prize in Medicine for their discovery of penicillin and its curative effect in various infectious diseases. Penicillin saved the lives of millions of World War II soldiers. After the war penicillin continued to be a successful healer of pneumonia, wounds, inflammation, and a wide spectrum of other sicknesses, and it brought back to health thousands of men, women, and children everywhere in the world.

However natural "antibiotics" had been known to folk healers, midwives, and "witches" for centuries.

Be smart! Start your own green clinic right in your house. Probably you already have in your house a good stocked "apothecary" with dried herbs and herbal teas. Now you can add something new and useful to that pharmacy.

Begin by buying aloe (*Aloe vera*) in a small pot. You can easily find it in a supermarket for about two dollars. Learn how to cherish this noble plant, whose motherland (or origin) is tropical Africa. *Aloe vera* was known to the Greeks and Romans, who used the gel for wounds. They carefully sliced it along the center of a leaf and peeled back the edges. Then using the blunt edge of a knife, they scraped the gel from the leaf.

Keep your potted aloe plant on the windowsill in the kitchen. Now if someone gets burned while in your house, you can help them with your plant. Prepare your first remedy in natural medicine by making aloe gel. It's easy and it takes only a few minutes. To soothe minor burns, scalds, or sunburn, cut off a fresh leaf from an *Aloe vera* plant. Split the leaf open and apply the thick gel to the affected area immediately. Since the safety of such treatment has never been questioned, this is a therapy you can offer to your family or friends as well as a treatment for dry skin, insect bites, and fungal infections.

And this is not all you can do. You can offer inhalation too. Use the gel in a steam inhalant for bronchial congestion. Bring to a boil three cups of water. Soak one *Aloe vera* leaf in the water for five minutes. The water will absorb the medicinal qualities of this plant. Then place your face over the boiling concoction, cover your head with a towel, and breathe in the steam. Use the Greeks' and Romans' method of preparation of aloe gel by carefully slicing the leaf along its center and peeling the edges. Then with the blunt edge of a knife, scrap the gel from the leaf. Put the gel into a pot with boiling water. If you find this method too complicated, just use the first one mentioned above because it is really easier to do. Split the aloe open. A thick gel will appear in the center of a leaf. Put a whole split leaf in a pot with boiling water. Let it steep for five minutes. Then cover your head with a towel and breathe as long as you can to relieve you bronchial or nasal congestion.

Do you know that extracts of aloe leaves were used once in some countries on children's fingers to stop nail-biting!?

Ancient Egyptians treated various inflammatory diseases with mold from barley grain. We now refer to this particular type of mold as tetracycline, an antibiotic with a wide spectrum of action.

When I was suffering with a bout of pneumonia, my doctor prescribed for me several different antibiotics because none in particular had an effect on me. My body was immune and refused to absorb the initial chemical treatments he had prescribed, and not until I was given tetracycline did my body respond and use it to heal the pneumonia.

Certain molds have proved their healing properties, but many other natural substances used in green medicine are not recognized by the medical community. Why? I believe one reason is that there has not been enough research conducted on them to earn the faith of the masses, so understandably skepticism prevails.

In ancient times people knew and understood the medicinal qualities of thousands of plants, trees, flowers, and stones—more so than we do now. Today these substances appear to most to be "exotic" or "preposterous" cures. And do you know why? Because modern doctors don't know much about them, and today's scientists are preoccupied with complicated "computer-led" researches in modern, sterile clean laboratories, where miraculous compounds are created daily. These compounds are the lucrative symbols of a powerful and very wealthy pharmaceutical industry.

It astounds me when I see this dismissing and ill-disposed attitude adopted by so many of our doctors and scientists. These are the professionals who are bound by their duties as health-care providers and researchers to be concerned with providing the best of care to their patients, and yet they disregard the knowledge of the past. They are obliged to review this knowledge and bring it back from the dust of centuries to be employed once again as a natural preventative and healing tool. There are in the world thousands of simple natural matters and means and thousands of ancient remedies that are awaiting research and distribution.

Thousands of natural substances are hidden in flora and fauna and in other treasures of Mother Nature, but yet they are still unknown to us.

Usually novice botanists consider all types of moss as peat moss. They confuse sphagnum (peat moss) with green downy which is like a tiny fir tree and is called "cuckoo flax" in Russia. This "cuckoo flax" has one small "box" on the "foot"—sporangium. The other kind is soft, bright-green branchy moss, which has several sporangiums.

A well-known Russian botanist and writer, Nikolai Verzilin, wrote in his book, *Follow Robinson*,[2] "Sphagnum, when it is wet is pale-green on top, and white on the bottom. It covers solidly the peat bog, usually where cranberries and cloud-berries grow."

In 1919, in a young Soviet Republic, a fierce fight raged in the north between the Russian tsar's white guards and the Red Army soldiers. There were many wounded Red Army soldiers, and the field hospital was running low on supplies of cotton/wool bandages and iodine. There was nothing else the hospital nurses could do but to cut underwear in narrow strips for bandages while old bandages were washed and dried. But cotton wool, an irreplaceable material for treating festering wounds, was not available.

When the supply of bandages and all dressing materials was depleted, the hospital doctors and nurses were forced to find an alternative. They had no means to obtain additional bandages and did not know what to use instead. Physicians were frustrated and distraught as they witnessed the soldiers suffering from wounds that were left unattended because of the lack of bandaging.

One physician decided to take a walk and think about the problem. Winter had just begun and the northern village where the hospital was located was bleak, grey, and gloomy. The trees stood naked in solemn silence waiting for a severe frost, which would surely be upon them any day.

The doctor arrived on the outskirts of the village to find a marsh covered with a first snow. The doctor became irritated and trampled down on the hummock. The situation appeared hopeless until he realized that he was standing atop clean, white moss sphagnum. Instantly he recalled that many years prior, during his student years in medical school, he had examined a leaf of sphagnum moss under a microscope and found large empty cells. He took a closer look at the moss under his feet now and saw frozen water in their empty cells. He knew that dried moss is used extensively by farmers to absorb dung water. The doctor immediately guessed that dried moss could be used successfully to absorb the liquids from festering wounds.

Unexpectedly this unknown Russian doctor had made a scientific discovery and found a substitute for cotton wool bandages. He was excited about his find and told the hospital staff about the white sphagnum moss.

The next morning a deep snow fell from the heavy gray sky. It became very cold, but it did not deter the hospital staff from their mission. All hospital attendants, stretcher-bearers, and nurses went to the marsh to collect sphagnum. They dug into the snow and removed almost 600 pounds of frozen layers of moss in less than three hours. The harvest was enough to keep the wounded soldiers swaddled in clean bandages through the severe winter.

To prepare the moss and adapt it to the needs of the patients, the moss was allowed to thaw. Then the water was squeezed from it and the sheets of moss were placed to dry on the floor of a warm room. In 24 hours it was ready to use as a substitute for the precious cotton wool.

It proved to be an effective bandaging material, but in addition sphagnum partially replaced the healing effects of iodine as well. Wounds dressed with the moss were noted to heal more rapidly because the moss contains a special disinfectant which is identical to carbolic acid and inhibits the growth of purulent bacteria.

When I was a child, my friends and I would tell spooky stories around the fire on our camping trips. My grandpa used to tell us horror stories that took place in marshy areas. He told us about ancient boats, wooden cabins and shacks, animal bones, and human skeletons that had been found in marshes. He told me about the body of a knight, suited in full heavy metal armor that had been found in a marsh.

His stories greatly affected me. I spent many sleepless nights trying to understand why a marsh is often such a sad, mysterious, and deadly place.

Scientist-botanists often find pieces of tree trunks and stems of thorny plants that have been perfectly preserved in peat for two hundred thousand years. How is this possible? The preservation action is caused by a vacuum created by the absence of air, the acidity of the marsh, and the disinfectant action of the sphagnum. These three conditions provide a safe place for these materials to remain perfectly preserved for a long time.

If you are curious by nature, conduct your own experiment with sphagnum. Place a piece of dry sphagnum in a glass jar with water and it will float on the surface like a cork.

To use sphagnum moss as bandaging material (don't laugh; you might find yourself on a camping trip miles from civilization wishing you had paid attention to this), the moss must be soaked with water, wrung out, and dried before being applied to the wound. Do not allow the moss to dry to a brittle state because it will compress and lose its ability to absorb liquid.

This little-known discovery made in pure desperation by a Russian doctor in 1919 can be developed today in research and perfected in preparation of natural materials for a treatment of wounds, ulcers, abscesses, inflammation, and burns.

It would likely be beneficial for our respected scientists to explore "the kitchens" of our grandmothers, midwives, and "witches." Unfortunately my walking "Green Encyclopedia," my grandma, has passed away, but I am thankful that my dear mother is alive, and she is there for me to consult regarding healing herbs and natural remedies. I consider myself the lucky heir to their extensive knowledge, which I began to document in a thick notebook when I was 12 years old. Day by day I recorded recipes and natural remedies that were passed down through the generations as treatments to prevent and fight disease.

I read many medical books from Mama's library and she shared with me her knowledge. I continue to consult with Mama, whose knowledge, even today, is extensive and focused on natural, effective, and harmless methods of green treatment. I have devoted my life to extensive research of the prescriptions and recipes of great ancient doctors.

Today traditional, modern, and alternative medicines can no longer go each in their own way. We must learn to use them in synthesis, drawing from the best of each to reach their common goal—to prevent and treat disease.

Avicenna, author of *The Canon of Medicine*, lived in Bukhara, Uzbekistan. In some encyclopedias Avicenna (Ibn-Sina; 980-1037) is represented as a Persian physician and philosopher. *The Canon of Medicine* is considered to be the greatest of all his prolific writing in theology, metaphysics, mathematics, and logic. It remained a standard medical text in Europe until the Renaissance.

Avicenna relied on his own discoveries and adopted remedies from his ancestors—great physicians of ancient Greece, India, China, Egypt, Sri Lanka, Indonesia, and Africa. He also borrowed the wisdom of healers. While some may argue that the research on which he based his methods was ancient and no longer plausible in our current age of advanced technology, there is wisdom in the methods he employed that cannot be overlooked today. It is our choice to use our own judgment.

Avicenna did not hold an "authority's" opinion above his own. He conducted his own experiments just as scientists do today. I do believe that he had more freedom to do as he wished than if he were employed by a powerful pharmaceutical company exploring the possibilities of the modern science of biochemistry. I sometimes imagine how Avicenna might function in today's sterile, white modern laboratories with their state-of-the-art computers.

He practiced nearly 40 years in the king's palaces, in the shacks of poor workers, and in farm houses. During this time he had practical experience in using and validating the effectiveness of natural remedies. He approached these folk "prescriptions" from a critical point of view. After much research, he explained the nature and influence of various remedies on the patients' physiology and illness.

Granted, as we read Avicenna's words today, they may seem primitive, but thousands of years from today so will the ideas of our current scholars, scientists, and physicians. There is truth in the old saying that "the new is well-forgotten old."

In an ancient Talmud it is written: "There is no leprous people and those suffering with pus in Babylon, because there the beets are eaten, the honey is drunken and people are washed with waters of the Euphrates." Thousands of years separate us from ancient times. Today researchers affirm that the population in Iraq, contemporary Iraqis, consume red beets in big quantities. And statistics tell us that occurrences of cancer are minimal. But in a span between those thousands of years ago and our current age, Galen, Dioscorides, Hippocrates, Avicenna, and many other skilled physicians of ancient times also knew about the medicinal properties of beets and used them as a natural healing medicine in treating diseases of intestinal properties and lymphatic glands, anemia, fever, nettle-rash, and putrid (putrefactive) and malignant sores.

Scientific studies have proven that the ancient doctors were correct in their evaluation of the effective medicinal properties of red beets. It was established that beets contain cellulose, apple, lemon, and other biogenetic acids which increase peristalsis of the intestines. Betaine in beets supports splitting (breaking up) and the adaptation of protein in food. Beets participate in the formation of choline, which increases the vitality of liver cells.

Recommended remedies using organic beets include:

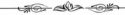

 1. Eat before breakfast three to five ounces of cooked beets if you suffer from chronic constipation, liver diseases, or indigestion.

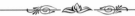

 2. As a highly nutritious supplement for anemia and as a means to improve metabolism, make ½ glass fresh beet juice and mix it with ½ glass fresh carrot or black radish juice.

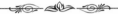

 3. Fresh beet juice mixed with two teaspoons honey makes a natural medicine for healing hypertension or acting as a calmative.

Beets contain relatively big quantities of iodine and magnesium, which make this vegetable "a must have" in daily nutrition for all ages, but especially for elderly people and those who suffer from atherosclerosis.

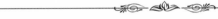

 4. Peel one or two organic red beets and cook until soft. Cool, grate, and add olive oil and thinly sliced almonds. Mix and eat the salad as breakfast, lunch, or appetizer.

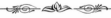

5. Cut two small pieces of raw organic red beet. Put in nostrils and beet will heal catarrh, a head cold, or sinus problems.

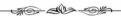

 6. Grate a raw organic red beet and apply to a sore (ulcer) or tumors. It supports the healing process naturally.

 7. Grate a raw organic red beet. Put between two layers of cheesecloth. Apply to the anus for 15 minutes. This is one of the best natural treatments for hemorrhoids.

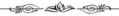

But the best kept secret of red beets is their ability to prevent and treat tumors, in addition to diuretic, laxative, anti-inflammatory and pain reducing benefits. Grandma once had problems with her liver. She instinctually began to eat salads with grated raw, red beets, sprinkled with lemon juice and sunflower oil. After two months her liver problems disappeared. She tried to "recruit" us to eat her salads, but no one in our family signed up for it. So, Grandma said, "If you don't understand how to keep yourself healthy and prevent illnesses, I'll show you!" And, indeed she did! She found other ways to entice us to eat red beets. I am not referring to borscht, which was already on her menu as our favorite meal. Following up on her beliefs about health benefits of beets, she invented and often created for us fresh beet juice and two absolutely fabulous salads, which she called "Red Wheels."

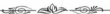

 8. Cook two medium organic red beets (skin on) in two cups water until soft. Cool, peel and grate them. In a bowl, combine the beets with two cloves crushed garlic, two tablespoons chopped walnuts and a pinch of salt. Add two tablespoons organic nonfat sour cream, vegetable mayonnaise or olive oil. Mix the salad and enjoy!

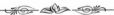

 9. Herring under a fancy red beet coat. Place herring fillets on a plate and cover with a layer of cooked and grated beets, a layer of chopped walnuts or pine nuts, then a layer of diced red onion and chopped parsley. Sprinkle with pomegranate juice. If you prefer, use grated raw beets instead of cooked beets. Herring offers additional benefits in combination with beets; it helps to treat headaches and fatigue.

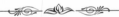

One day I asked Grandma why she craved her raw red beet salads. She said that when she began to have problems with her liver, she had a "call and request" from her body for red beets. In reality, the sick cells in her body, especially in her liver, made an independent, and obviously a smart decision for her by determining what she was lacking and what was needed. Grandma was healed by the vitamins and nutrients in raw, red beets. You see our cells know better and help us to treat our bodies in a natural way. The badger had the same experience. He felt that he needed the stump mold to heal his wounds.

My Grandma was not alone in her findings. She was one of hundreds of others who experienced an inner understanding of what kind of plant, vegetable, or fruit their body and cells, affected by illness, needed the most and they healed themselves with it. They passed the valuable information to others, who lacked the ability to feel it. These plants, vegetables, fruits, and flowers then became basic medicines of an ancient green pharmacy.

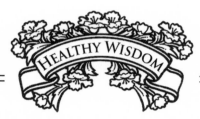

Small children–small worries, big children–big worries.

—*Russian saying*

My grandmother sits in a chair near our big lilac bush blossoming with delicate, fragrant, purple flowers. She tells me and my sister a beautiful tale about the grapevine of happiness, which can help to keep you healthy or heal you when you are sick. I'll remember this story forever because it was told by you, Grandma.

—*S. K.*

The sea possesses a power over one's moods that has the effect of a will. The sea can hypnotize. Nature in general can do so.

—*Henrik Ibsen (1828–1906), Norwegian poet and playwright*

Chapter 3

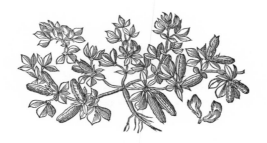

A Healthy Spirit Lives in
a Healthy Body

Think of our life in Nature—daily to be shown matter,
to come in contact with it, rocks, trees, wind on our cheeks!
The solid earth! The actual world! The common sense!
Contact! Contact! Who are we? Where are we?

—Henry David Thoreau (1817-1862), American writer

FACTS

In 2000 Americans enjoyed the longest life expectancy in U.S. history—almost 77 years, based on preliminary figures. The life expectancy of men was 74 years and for women almost 80 years. A century earlier, life expectancy was 48 years for men and 51 years for women.[3]

At the same time 3 in 5 adults ages 20–74 are overweight. One in four Americans is considered obese. Almost 40 percent engage in no physical activity during leisure time, and women are more sedentary than men. One in 10 Americans ages 45–54, 1 in 5 of those 55–64 years, 1 in 4 of those 65–74 years, and 1 in 3 of those 75 years and over, report being in fair or poor health.

The same report noted that Americans spent $1.3 trillion on healthcare in 2000, or 13.2 percent of the gross domestic product, far more than any other nation. A third of the health-care dollar was spent on hospital care, about ⅕ on physicians, and almost ⅒ on prescription drugs. The cost of prescription drugs increased 15 percent a year from 1995 to 2000—faster than any other category of spending.[4]

Healthy People 2010[5]—the nation's health agenda for the first decade of the twenty-first century—indicates that differences in life expectancy between populations suggest a substantial need and opportunity for improvement: "At least 18 countries with a population of 1 million or more have life expectancies greater than the United States for both men and women."

"Chapter Goal 1: Increase Quality and Years of Healthy Life" states, "However, quality of life reflects a general sense of happiness and satisfaction with our lives and environment. General quality of life, including health, recreation, culture, rights, values, beliefs, aspirations, and the conditions that support a life containing these elements."[6] We can only hope that the nation's health agenda for the first 10 years of the twenty-first century will work. But what will happen if it does not work? Keep yourself updated!

A suburb of the Russian tsar's huge empire, former Bessarabia, now Moldova, holds many warm memories of my childhood and my home. I remember the hilly countryside with its sunny vineyards, fields with blossoming herbs and flowers, and big, sometimes giant, walnut trees everywhere. A golden and unforgettable time of my happy childhood was spent in our beautiful home there.

Our big house on a hill was built of thick beech logs. It was cool in summer and warm in the winter. It was filled with love and kindness, our family often including grandparents from my mother's and father's sides; folk wisdom; and the aroma of grapes, walnuts, herbs, and wildflowers.

Within our home in the country was a most magical place—the basement. Grandma's and Grandpa's homemade libations and elixirs shared that space. There Grandpa stored wooden barrels filled with his homemade crystal-clear white and rosé wines and lined shelf upon shelf with old-fashioned European glass bottles containing liquors and cognacs that he carefully prepared each fall.

In another part of the basement Grandma filled her beautiful and simple European glass bottles with her homemade natural medicine recipes; tinctures of herbs, berries or fruits; and aromatic oils. On special racks in autumn she would hang handmade "necklaces" strung with dried fruits and herbs, or *Vitachella* with nuts, which we called "grape sausage." Her secret recipe for

Vitachella included cooked grape juice with special spices and, of course, walnuts. From November to May we enjoyed these dainty tidbits full of a variety of natural ingredients and vitamins. My sister and I were allowed to go anytime to the basement, which we called our "Sweet Fairyland," to tear down and eat a grape "necklace."

Another room of the basement was stocked with herbs. Some were suspended from the ceiling; others were carefully wrapped and packed in parchment. Near this herbarium was Grandma's and Mama's laboratory where they prepared their miraculous natural medicines for our family, for our friends and neighbors, and for Mama's patients.

Grandma and Mama never sold their natural medicines. They were old-fashioned women. They shared a strong belief that if the medicines were sold, they would lose their ability to heal. Instead they felt they must offer them mercifully and free of charge to those who needed them. This mission of mercy helped many people overcome their illnesses. Because we grew up in a society without mass-produced and heavily marketed antibiotics and drugs, we, as the ancient Greeks, developed a strong, natural foundation in our bodies to be healthy human beings.

Once upon a time there lived an old man in the sunny Valley of Roses. Long ago he planted a big vineyard, which brought him a rich bounty year after year. The vineyard was his passion, and so he decided to build a beautiful big house right in the center of it.

Over time the house became entwined in grapevines. He believed that grapes and their vines would defend his hearth from evil people, from dust, and from the harmful effects of a hot, dry summer. He also believed that his mighty grapevines would clean and refresh the air. Overall his grapevines, he believed, would make his life peaceful and healthy.

Grapes and vines are symbols of well-being, friendship, and attachment. Like the pineapple, they are a symbol of welcome. When the old man's grapevines blossomed in June, he would drop to his knees, press his nose into the lush grape-laden vines, and breathe in their delicate aroma.

He waited patiently for September to come, when he would harvest great quantities of ripe amber, ruby, and rose grapes swollen with sweet juice. With his face illuminated by the brightest smile and his eyes shining with sparks of happiness, he would begin his task of creating "Sunny Beams" juices and wines. The old man went about his work in a passionate way and often said that he was so happy he felt as if he could kiss everyone in the whole world a thousand times.

This man was my grandfather.

Now I will share a story that he shared with me when I was a little girl.

"Come here, into the vineyard" he told his children one day. "The grapevine will pass happiness along to you too." The children came many times to his purple and green kingdom, sparkling with millions of thin, almost invisible luminescent threads of sun rays and he told them everything he knew about grapevines and happiness.

The grapevine has always inspired great artists and poets. Many centuries ago a Greek artist painted a grapevine that became a famous legend. The grapes he painted were so attractive and realistic on the canvas that the birds mistakenly thought they could eat them. They flocked to the painting from everywhere to take a bite of happiness and enjoy the taste of juicy grapes. But the birds soon learned that the talented artist had fooled them.

"So don't be mistaken in your life," Grandpa told us. "See things as they really are. Don't fool yourself. Whatever you do, do it well and you will always be satisfied with yourself and happy with the whole world. It's so easy. If you do not do a good job, you will have to pay the consequences. You will have to correct what you did wrong and do it over and over again and you will not come to a great result. My advice to you is to do everything right in the first place and all good things will come back to you like a boomerang."

Grandpa used to say. "The land, especially the vineyard, loves hard workers and happy people. If you are in a fine mood, your grapevines will be too. Your feelings are passed along to them." My grandfather worked hard every day from sunrise to sunset with his brothers by his side. This was the way in which he lived his life and he accepted it and was satisfied with it. He never wished to change it. In the 1930s the brothers built a family empire: vineyards, orchards, fields. They built a plant where they made their fine wines and juices.

Then the Soviets came in 1940 and they nationalized people's private properties. They prohibited private citizens from owning commercial vineyards and orchards. The two oldest brothers fled to France and Canada. For a year after that, my grandfather could not recover from the shock of what the Soviets had done or the loneliness he felt without his brothers, nor could he adjust to his new life without his beloved vineyard and orchard. He became terribly sick for a long time, suffering from shock and distress.

One day my father gave him hope and renewed energy. He got permission for Grandpa to grow his cherished grapes and fruits on one acre of land in the outskirts of the city in which we lived. And Grandpa planted with great enthusiasm his new and last vineyard. He was always a gentle and kind man who didn't talk much. I never heard him complain of being tired.

I watched him toil in his orchard, and it was for me a priceless lesson because I learned how happy a man could be doing what he loved to do. I recalled many times the story of my grandfather who began his life anew after losing everything. Grandpa, this tiny but strong man with the soul of a child, had never been ill in his life. But the magic of our human nature is that we can adjust to any changes in our lives. Positive ones we adjust to in the blink of an eye; the negative changes take longer. The main point is that we can get accustomed to almost everything—if we *love* and *believe*.

Grandpa quickly became accustomed to his new life and a much smaller piece of land, and again he was happy, healthy, optimistic, and cheerful. He could not imagine life without his work. He couldn't imagine losing his liaison with Nature and the vineyard. It was his magical world of the grapevines of happiness. As long as he dwelled in this spot, he was healthy and happy.

"A healthy spirit lives in a healthy body" is a wise expression attributed to the ancient Greeks. They did not have antibiotics or other chemical stimulators, such as sedative drugs, which so many people use now—and yet they were healthy and happy.

We must maintain our health and energy to keep up with the fast pace of life in the twenty-first century. Unfortunately too many people are unaware that they are poisoning their bodies with chemicals in an effort to obtain rapid relief from their ailments.

While our physical health is supremely important, we cannot neglect our mental and emotional health either. Most of us, in an effort to manage our jobs, home life, and other roles we have taken on, must process a seemingly endless and continuous stream of information flying at us at breakneck speed via our modern media. Consequently we become overstressed and quickly burn out.

Stress has been recognized as the major contributor to many neuroses and cardio-vascular problems. Scientists say that one in three people suffer from a nervous disorder or other form of stress-related disease. We must remember to establish boundaries for ourselves to maintain a healthy balance of work and play. Moderation is the key. Are we operating within our physical and intellectual limits? Have we succumbed to weakness and vulnerability? Or have we learned to accumulate and sustain reserves of our energy? We must all learn to tap into our reservoirs of strength and energy and keep them effective for as long as we can. How?

To maintain our health and conserve our energy, we must identify and eliminate the bad habits we practice that deplete them. First, we can temper our use of over-the-counter chemical preparations which are widely and readily available in drug stores. Taken over the years, they rob us of our strength, poison us, and destroy our internal organs.

Chemical drugs such as sedatives and stimulants may give us initial relief, but for a short time only. The body's response to them often varies or changes. The little pill you popped a few months ago to take the edge off or put you to sleep may now make you nervous, dizzy, or prone to insomnia or cause other adverse side effects.

Prescription drugs used to treat illnesses such as heart disease, high blood pressure, thyroid disease, and diabetes should not be used for the long term, but only in the heat of our illness or during our recovery, and always under the supervision of a physician. If you become concerned about the amount of medicine you are taking or the duration of a course of drug therapy, ask your doctor about herbal alternatives.

Several years ago I read an article, "Doctors Are the Third Leading Cause of Death in the U.S., Causing 250,000 Deaths Every Year." It was published in the largest and the most respected medical journal in the world, the *Journal of the American Medical Association.*[7]

I remember getting a feeling of desperation after reading this article. None of the wire services picked up this story; the news media let it slip by. Perhaps the publishers decided that an article documenting the tragedy of the traditional medical paradigm of the United States might cause several million readers to rise up and ask questions.

When I mentioned this article to one of my friends, a journalist and breast cancer survivor, she said, "I think that this number, 250,000, is even higher now." The author, Dr. Barbara Starfield of the John Hopkins School of Hygiene and Public Health, described how the U.S. health-care system may *contribute* to poor health. The figure, 250,000 deaths per year, is comprised of so-called iatrogenic cases! This term is defined as "induced in a patient by a physician's activity, manner or therapy."

Another analysis concluded that consecutive patients experience negative effects in outpatient settings with 116 million extra physician visits, 17 million extra prescriptions, 17 million hospitalizations, 3 million long-term hospital admissions, 199,000 additional deaths, and $77 billion in extra costs.

However, evidence from a few studies indicated that as many as 20 to 30 percent of patients receive inappropriate care. The poor performance of the United States was recently confirmed by the World Health Organization, which used different data and ranked the United States 15th among 25 industrialized countries in healthcare. In any case 250,000 deaths per year from iatrogenic causes constitute the third leading cause of death in the United States, after deaths from heart disease and cancer. Shocking news, isn't it?

We know that every doctor graduating from medical school takes the Hippocratic Oath to treat people no matter what. Doctors make a sacred promise "to do no harm," but statistics show that doctors and hospitals *do* make mistakes. Another report that I found shocking was from the Institute of Medicine. It showed that medical mistakes are a common and potentially life-threatening risk.

Dr. Joseph Mercola, from the Optimal Wellness Center in Shaumburg, Illinois, had this to say about it in his newsletter: "It is an intolerable situation, especially when it's taking place in the United States, which leads the world in medical advances."[8]

So what are we waiting for? Our ancestors survived by being smart and keeping themselves healthy with help from Mother Nature. Most of us come into this world as healthy human beings. Our bodies are designed to maintain the best in us. We are built to be solid, strong, and energetic. We can keep our bodies free of toxins and cleanse our systems periodically with herbs such as burdock, chamomile, dandelion, and garlic. Our natural resources, such as the sun, earth, and Nature, provide us with optimal energy. Thus we are perfectly capable to self-heal when we are sick or injured.

We are intended to live a long and healthy life, but only on one condition: we must take our health into our hands and maintain the knowledge of how to do that. We are our own best friends. So take good care of your best friend. By knowing the curative and preventative qualities of herbs and plants, we can safely treat our ailments and prevent further diseases, weaknesses, or hopelessness from wreaking havoc in our lives.

We must take control of our health *while we are still healthy*. Medical research organizations are not proponents of preventative medicine because their work is based on illness.

"There is no money to be made from healthy people." This statement is excerpted from an article, "The Life That Is Costing Hundreds of Billions of Dollars," published by a health organization in New Zealand.[9] "This is why the medical and research establishments are not in the least interested in prevention (practically all diseases are preventable)."

Preventive care *is* the solution to disease. It can keep us healthy and free of illnesses. We can do it! We just have to learn *how* to do it.

How can we begin to think differently about how we maintain our healthy bodies and help prevent serious illness? First, get smart! Keep up to date on the latest research on alternative health measures. We must equip ourselves with this powerful tool. With knowledge we can provide first aid and preventive healthcare in our own homes for ourselves and our families and avoid spending a fortune on doctor visits and drugstore prescriptions.

Greek mythology tells us that Apollo, the god of prophesy, music, and healing, equated the medicinal worth of the common garden radish to that of gold, rapeseed to silver, and turnip to lead. Apollo later fathered a son, Asclepiad (Roman, Aesculapius), who is known to us now as the ancient Greek god of medicine and healing.

Aesculapius in Roman mythology is a god of healing. His name became synonymous with "doctor" or "healer" in an ironically playful way. Aesculapius or Asclepiad is known as the god of healing who became so skilled that he attempted to resurrect the dead, thus angering Zeus, who struck him dead with a thunderbolt.

The medical profession has adopted his symbol, a staff entwined by a snake.

I know some great American and European doctors who not only employ the use of well-known antibiotics and other drugs under their strict supervision, but they also prescribe and make their own healing herbal remedies. They garnered these natural remedies from centuries of wisdom, proven by generations of healers in Europe, Asia, and North and South America. They know that their patients rely on their knowledge and attitude. Good doctors are compelled to gain victory over disease.

Popping an over-the-counter pain tablet may provide temporary relief from a simple headache, but most of these drugs will not provide relief for migraine headaches—and loading up on chemicals over long periods of time does the body little good. Why not try a natural remedy instead?

Not everyone knows that most of us have in our kitchens a well-stocked "apothecary." Even today the common garden radish, swede, and turnip are valued in folk medicine for their healing properties.

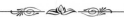

 1. One tablespoon of garden radish juice, squeezed from the root and taken three times, is helpful in decreasing coughs and soothing a hoarse voice. It is useful in treating dysfunctions of the liver and gall bladder, including the formation of stones in the kidneys and liver.

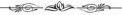

 2. Garden radish juice makes an excellent massage emollient in the treatment of rheumatism and colds.

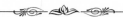

 3. Although in most cases not as effective as radish juice, the juice of a turnip mixed with honey settles a cough.

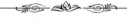

 4. Cooked and pulverized turnip root used as a plaster helps heal gout in the foot.

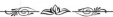

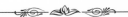

5. A plaster of washed, fresh cabbage leaves applied to the forehead and temples relieves headaches.

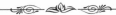

6. Try the same plaster to soothe a burn, bruise, or external abrasions.

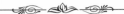

7. Systematically chew sauerkraut to make weak gums stronger.

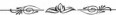

8. A wart rubbed with the fresh juice of sour apples over 10 days will darken, decrease in size, and then disappear.

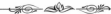

9. One tablespoon each of rum, glycerin, and lemon juice mixed and rubbed into the scalp strengthens the hair.

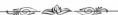

10. A cotton pad soaked in the freshly squeezed juice of two to three garlic cloves or one cut garlic clove rubbed onto the affected area treats skin disorders, including eczema and balding. Garlic acts as an effective antiseptic, antibacterial, and antifungal healer for other infected skin conditions such as acne.

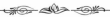

11. Drink ½ cup of freshly squeezed cabbage juice 30 minutes before breakfast, lunch, and dinner for three to four weeks to help with weight loss.

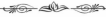

12. A freshly grated beet, mixed with one tablespoon sour cream, is used to treat acne and purulent (festering) pimples by applying to the affected area for five minutes.

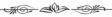

13. Strong black coffee made with freshly ground coffee beans can be used as a hand bath and to treat nail fungus.

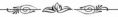

14. Painful corns can be treated by rubbing them with fresh tomato slices for 15 minutes a day for two weeks.

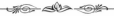

In your kitchen you will most likely find a vegetable that sailors have used for ages to treat burns, stomach ailments, and scurvy while navigating the high seas—the potato.

Potato (*Solanum*) is a perennial plant. In many countries it is "second bread." It is almost impossible to find another plant that is so similar to the simple bread we eat every day. As a main food product, the potato is also one of the favorites in "people's medicine," and it can usually be found right in our pantries.

Potato is a diuretic, and if cooked, can successfully treat respiratory diseases. The following remedies are best when used with organic potatoes.

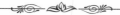

15. Cook two to three potatoes in water. Drain. Dice potatoes and keep in the same pot. Cover your head with a towel and breathe in the potato steam for 10 minutes. Repeat the same procedure three to four times every two to three hours to ease breathing.

The potato is called in Italy *tartufolli* or "devil's apple." The potato came to Europe about four centuries ago when Pedro Cieza de Leon, 13, stowed away aboard a ship of Spanish sailors, who were to be the first conquerors of South America. He eventually found himself together with them in a wonderful country called Peru. While Spanish soldiers searched for gold, killed the Peruvians, and burned their homes, little Pedro was mesmerized by the people of Peru. Their strange-looking buildings and well-made furnishings fascinated him. He wanted to learn more about the lifestyles of the bronzed inhabitants of Peru, so he wrote down everything he saw.

In 1553 in the Spanish city of Seville, he published the *Chronica del Perú*. In this book we find his early reference to the potato. He wrote, "Pappa is a special kind of ground nut. It becomes soft when cooked, like a baked chestnut with skin no thicker than a truffle (mushroom)."

Spanish sailors were the first to try potatoes. Later the potato made its way to Italy, where the Peruvian *pappa* was renamed *tartufolli*. From there it gravitated to other countries.

By the end of the eighteenth century women in France were obsessed with the potato as a design accessory. They made potato flower bouquets and decorated their hair with single blooms. The popularity of potato flowers was booming. It seemed that there were not enough to go around, and people begin making artificial potato flowers. Only at the beginning of the nineteenth century did French farmers begin to cultivate potatoes for food under the enthusiastic support and promotion of French pharmacist, Antoine Parmantié.

Around the same time the potato flower became a favorite in Germany and was planted in flowerbeds adorning palaces. More than a hundred years ago a Russian tsar gave an order to farmers to cultivate potatoes. This order provoked so-called potato rebellions because Russian farmers did not want to plant the "devil's apple." But today the potato is popular in Russia, as it is everywhere in the world. Each nation considers it as their own native plant.

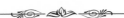

 16. Potato in a Dress Uniform. Wash a potato well and bake it in its skin. Cook one beet in water until soft. Peel the skin off both vegetables. Mince the beet and mix with the potato flesh and with one teaspoon olive oil or sour cream. Then eat it. It helps to reduce high blood pressure.

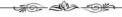

 17. Wash one organic potato and dry. Make a fresh juice in a juicer from this potato and its skin. Drink it to normalize stomach acidity and to regulate the digestive system. It will also treat stomach and intestinal cramps. Potato juice is also helpful in treating heartburn, dizziness, and vomiting.

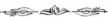

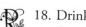

 18. Drink ¾ cup fresh potato juice before breakfast. Then lie down for 30 minutes. You can eat one hour later. Do it for 10 days, then take a break for 10 days. Continue the same procedure for another 10 days.

Fresh potato juice helps people with duodenal ulcers and stomach and gastritis problems.

 19. Fresh organic potato juice is a well-known recipe in folk medicine for treating headaches. Take ¼ cup potato juice two times a day—in the morning before breakfast and before you go to bed.

Fresh organic potato juice helps those suffering from tuberculosis. European scientists confirmed that the potato contains a highly valuable substance—tuberose, which destroys micro-bacteria and combats tuberculosis. The Latin name for potato is *Solanum tuberosum*.

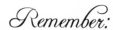 *Remember:*

Try these remedies under the supervision of your physician. You should use fresh potato juice at once. Never store it. Make fresh juice as needed.

 20. As a preventive measure, people with stomach and duodenal ulcers can drink fresh potato juice twice a year—in the spring and in the fall. Take ¼ cup potato juice two times a day before meals for two weeks. Make a fresh portion every day.

 21. Raw potato helps to treat hemorrhoids (piles). Cut in a tubular shape and use as a suppository at night.

22. Peel the skin of one raw potato, cut the potato into chunks, cover with water, and cook without salt in an enamel pot. When the potato is soft, strain through a nylon sieve into a teacup and drink ½ cup or one tablespoon of the concoction three times a day. This is a good home remedy for treating a sore throat or a cold.

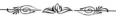

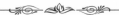

 23. Wash one organic potato and chop with its skin in a food processor for a few seconds. Spread potato poultice on the affected area. Apply three layers of gauze or cotton strips to hold the poultice in place for two hours. This potato compress is an effective anti-inflammatory healer. It helps to treat eczema, painful corns, and acute dermatitis. These compresses can be used every two hours several times a day.

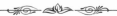

 24. Mix one teaspoon honey to ½ cup potato poultice and use as in #23.

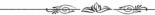

 25. Make ½ cup fresh organic potato juice mixed with honey as in #23. Soak a gauze napkin in it and apply it to the affected area. Honey is a valuable ingredient with its nutritional and anti-inflammatory properties.

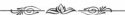

 26. Put slices of raw potato on eczema sores to soften and heal them.

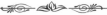

 27. Make a nutritious mask for dry, inflamed facial skin that is sensitive to dermatitis. Cook one potato, skinned and chopped, until soft. Crush it and whip with one tablespoon sour cream or two tablespoons skim milk. Apply to your face for 15 minutes. Wash it off. Look in the mirror. Your skin will be soft and glowing.

While potato flowers can be pretty accessories for women, they are a natural medicine as well. The wisdom of folk medicine found the use of them in a treatment of cancerous tumors. See #28.

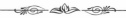

 28. Wash potato flowers and dry outdoors, out of the sun. Add one tablespoon dried flowers to one pint boiling water. Simmer for two to three hours on a hot stove. Drink ½ cup three times a day 30 minutes before meals. Do not consume more than four quarts of potato infusion per treatment, each of which lasts a week. Repeat three to four times a year.

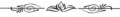

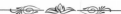

 29. Potato starch is also a good anti-inflammatory remedy. Use it instead of a powder to treat sensitive skin.

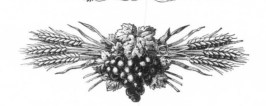

Grapes

There's no doubt that the potato is a great healer. Now let us look at the wonders that grapes can work.

Let me tell you what I learned in my childhood about these miraculous berries. One warm evening in June my sister and I were sitting on our porch with our grandma, looking at the grapevines and big oak trees that bordered it. The grapevines found these green giant oak trees to be a comfortable resting place. They climbed up to the top of the tallest oaks and then dropped from the summits to the ground. They looked different there than in our vineyard. These vines were like big mysterious and strange lianas that looked as if they belonged in a distant tropical paradise somewhere on an island in the Atlantic Ocean.

Grandma, who had finished her errands and assumed Grandfather's place on the porch to enjoy a quiet evening telling us the rich, colorful stories she loved so much, broke the silence. "Now we'll open again our pot of gold. Are you ready?" Grandma asked us.

What she called our "pot of gold" was simply her endless collection of unforgettable fairy tales. Grandma had a rare gift for infusing a special force into ordinary things or creatures surround us. I never had my fill of her stories and I was afraid that one day she would deplete her storehouse of fairy tales. But she always assured me that I should not be worried; she still had plenty of them from different parts of the world.

She could look at the smallest flower or animal and then tell stories about their lives. She wove a story as if she were tatting beautiful lace—a mix of fantasy, charm, and wisdom. Her stories became for me a way to see the world and to learn about it.

"Today, girls, I'll tell you the story about how the grapevine was born," Grandma began.

Once upon a time when the Sun and Earth were young, they were good friends. On the day when they both became 18 years old, they married. Nine months of their happy marriage passed quickly and their daughter was born—a grapevine. They gave her the name Ampelos, which means "grape" in Greek.

The Sun-father caressed Ampelos with his shining warm rays and washed her with sparkling and refreshing rains. Her mother, Earth, fed her generously with vital juices from the flowers, herbs, and trees. She grew up fast and became a tall, slender beauty.

She gave her parents millions of smiles and small grandchildren—grape berries. They appeared on a vine and ripened before the sunrise came. The first small berries blushed all over with the pale pink glow of the morning dawn. People in the village had never seen such a miracle in their lives. They came from all over to see it. Some approached the vines and tasted the berries. People liked them so much that they ate them all at once, but the vines did not stop growing and miraculously grapes appeared again and ripened again in just about six hours one day.

People were truly amazed. They observed how the grapes drank the gold juice made by the midday sun. They gathered a second time at the rich harvest and ate it all. After that, the grapevine stood empty. She had given everything she had to the people. But blessed by Sun and by Earth, Ampelos came up again in the late evening with new deep-blue and navy-black berries, which took the color of the southern night.

From this day on, Mother Nature gave the small children of the grapevine a generous gift of all colors that you can imagine: red, orange, yellow, green, blue, navy, purple, and pink. And Nature made the grapevine the only plant in the world with berries that are painted with all colors of the rainbow.

"Tomorrow," promised Grandma, "we'll go to the vineyard and you'll see how some grapes have all shades of white, green, and yellow and then turn into an amber warmth or golden gleam. It happens because the sun pours into each berry its bright colors, like foggy-grey, purple, and brown, and it makes sure that all grapes shine and brighten up under his radiant beams."

The grape was known for its effective healing properties 5,500 years ago in ancient Babylon and Mesopotamia. In 1613 this plant was brought to Russia and became very popular there. The grapevine gloriously conquered the hearts of the people around the world from time immemorial and it was recognized as highly nutritious and medicinal.

Today's biochemists affirm that 100-percent natural grape juice is equal in value to mother's milk. Grapes contain calcium, potassium, carotene, magnesium, manganese, glucose, pectin, and natural vitamins, such as C (ascorbic acid), B1 (thiamine), B6 (pyridoxine), B12 (cobalamin), dietary fiber, and organic acids, which are biological and nutritious stimulants. The human body will not function properly without them.

However people began to cultivate grapevines even earlier, about nine thousand years ago. They loved and nurtured this generous plant, producing "the berries of life." The grape was also called a wise plant and an immortal fruit. Grapes love the sun, so they were named "sunny berries."

In ancient times the grape was used as a tonic and effective diuretic, laxative, and expectorant. The grape is a great healer of a wide spectrum of illnesses when caught in the initial stage, such as bronchial asthma; pleurisy; tuberculosis; metabolism disorders; chronic inflammations of the alimentary canal; hemorrhoids; cardiovascular, liver, and kidney diseases; depression; arthritis; collapse/breakdown; and loss of blood.

The grape's sugar—glucose—is a strong antidote when poisoning by toxic substances such as morphine, arsenic, strychnine, and nitrate sodium has occurred.

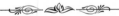

 30. Drink ½ cup freshly pressed grape juice a day for one month to maintain your normal weight. Grape juice is also helpful as a restorative remedy for the nervous system to heal anxiety and tension associated with excessive stress. As we know, excessive stress can lead to a variety of health problems, such as emotional instability (tendency to cry or be irritated for no obvious reason), inability to relax, palpitations, insomnia, or headaches. Fresh grape juice also improves the exchange of water and salt in the body and acts as a good antiseptic to clean harmful products, such as uric acid, from the system. And this is not all: Fresh grapes can prevent the formation of stones and sand in the urinary tract.

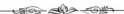

 31. Make "Baby Vinegar" using young green grapes. Fill a glass jar with two ounces of grapes. Add two tablespoons apple cider vinegar and one cup spring water. Simmer for two hours. Take one to two teaspoons daily before meals if you experience pains in joints and muscles or suffer from rheumatism. Store "Baby Vinegar" in the refrigerator.

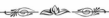

 32. Eat one ounce dried raisins, one ounce almonds or four to five walnuts, and two to three thin pieces of cheese (about an ounce) once a week for one month. Drink a cup of natural white grape juice once a week. It will make your heart muscle stronger, strengthen the nervous system, and relieve nervous headaches.

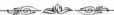

 33. As a remedy for fatigue, take ½ cup fresh grape juice a day. Two tablespoons every two hours is also very helpful as a preventive measure for a loss of energy, insomnia and depression, lack of determination, anger, or emptiness.

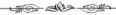

I believe that grapeseed extract—a heavily marketed product—should **not** be substituted for grapes and grape juices. It is extracted from the seeds of grapes (*Vitis vinifera)* and is combined with pine bark, which comes from the bark of the European coastal pine tree (*Pinus maritime* and *Pinus nigra*).

In *The Complete Guide to Herbal Medicines*[10], Charles W. Fetrow, Pharm. D., and Juan R. Avila, Pharm.D., wrote that grapeseed and pine bark "contain proanthocyanidins, a chemical marketed as Pycnogenol." It comes in tablets and capsules to treat cancer, inflammation, poor circulation, and varicose veins. The two pharmacists point out that products containing grapeseed and pine bark are sold under such names as Mega Juice, NutraPack, and Pycnogenol.

"The research shows," they indicate, "that although grape seed extract is popular in Europe, it hasn't been studied adequately in people for medical experts to recommend its medicinal use. The same holds true for pine bark."

I grew up in a family of European winemakers, but I never heard that any efficient grapeseed extract can be produced from grape seeds. However Mama made the best grapeseed oil I ever had. It was fresh from our winery and soft as velvet. It was much lighter to the touch than apricot kernel, almond, wheat germ, evening primrose, calendula, or rose hip oils. Mama kept it in tightly sealed European dark glass bottles.

I could see its emerald green spark even through these amber bottles. It was Mama's favorite oil for massaging. Sometimes she gave me a full body massage "to wake up my blood vessels" and increase the circulation of my blood and lymph system. Her skillful massage was a blessing, soothing my nervous system while her strong fingers glided effortlessly over my body, slick with her favorite grapeseed oil.

I have seen grapeseed oil for sale in bulk in health-food stores and recommended for use in cooking. I didn't notice any limits placed on its use, but it does contain about 120 calories per tablespoon. That's a lot compared to other cooking oils, such as olive oil, and adding excessive amounts of grape seed oil to the family diet may bring a problem of gaining weight or even obesity, so you'll be better off using it for an effective massage.

Again, you might ask, what about grapeseed extract in tablets and capsules created by a "bio-genius" in some modern laboratory? If grape seeds are so useful for internal consumption, why do we spit them out? Why not just eat fresh grapes with seeds? Many people prefer to eat seedless grapes anyway. What does this mean? Are the grape seeds useless or harmful for digestion—even in powder form? Obviously they are useless because our body will not accept anything that is against its nature. Just recall that when we eat fresh grapes with seeds, we spit them out as not chewable or acceptable to our digestive system.

The scientific name is grape seed, and other names are used by scientists, such as Muscat, Red Wine Extract, or *Vitis vinifera*. In August 2004, the American Heart Association (AHA) published a scientific discovery warning that little evidence was found for the effectiveness of antioxidant vitamin supplements to prevent cardiovascular disease. While acknowledging the benefits of antioxidants, the scientists who prepared the AHA recommendation advise getting natural antioxidants from foods rather than from supplements. Additionally some evidence from animal studies suggests that very high doses of antioxidants such as those in grapeseed extract may actually increase damage from oxidation.[11]

Perhaps my statement is controversial, but, as you see, some scientists hold the same view too. Moreover, some side effects, risks, and interactions have been reported by participants in clinical studies of grapeseed extract. Side effects include dizziness, cough, headaches, and nausea. Due to limited information about its potential effects on babies or infants, pregnant and breast-feeding women should not take grapeseed extract. This product may increase the effects of drugs, herbs, antioxidants or health supplements, if you have a bleeding or clotting disorder or if you are taking medicine to prevent blood clots. Grapeseed has not been evaluated by the FDA for safety or potential risks and/or advantages of grapeseed may not be known. Additionally there are no regulated manufacturing standards in place for these compounds. There have been instances where herbal/health supplements have been sold which were contaminated with toxic metals or other drugs.[12]

There are endless studies across the globe, including seven leading universities in Europe, that demonstrate the many benefits of grapeseed extract in fighting against free radicals in the body. This extensive research came in the late twentieth century from a so-called "French paradox." It was stated that the French had very low rates of heart disease and are not overweight while some of their diet and other factors, such as smoking and relatively late dinners, would be thought to contribute to higher incidences of heart or other diseases. Scientists believed the secret was in their regular consumption of red wines, which contain OPC (oligomeric proanthocyanidins). These antioxidants help to protect cells from free radical damage and promote healthy blood circulation and cardiovascular health.[13]

So why should we take grapeseed extract in tablets and capsules when we can enjoy fresh grapes, drink fresh grape juice, and get a gentle, natural treatment? Do not forget: Fresh sweet grapes are a generous gift of Nature. I was recently in France, and I observed how many people in Paris were eating dinner at 7–8 p.m. in restaurants. Numerous eateries there are crowded seven days a week. Usually visitors come in groups of 4 to 10 people. They order a very popular meal variety, which contains three pieces of meat and fish accompanied by mashed potatoes and vegetables and a bottle of red wine. Then they order fresh fruits and deserts, like famous crème brûlée, studded with bits of caramelized sugar, and French vanilla ice cream that has a custard base rich with egg yolks. And they are people of perfectly normal weight. I guess the secret of their diet is red wine; fresh grapes; and a slow, enjoyable consumption of good food while they socialize and have a pleasant conversation, adding positive emotions and vital energy overall.

An old expression says that "a new is an old that was well forgotten." The grapevine is registered as the oldest plant in the world. I first heard this fact in a lovely tale told by my grandmother.

In the evening the spicy aroma of a mélange of fruits and flowers permeated our southern garden. We sat in the gazebo in the middle of our garden and Grandma said, "Look at the star above you. This is the star of a boy named Ampel. Before he got to the sky, he lived on the earth."

The sky was shining with millions of silver stars, but one star radiated with all seven colors of the rainbow: purple and green, yellow and white, blue, red and orange. One bright star was hanging separately from the others as if it were in its special place. The star was Vindemiatrix (grape) and is located in the constellation of Virgo. It is easy to find on any map of the stars. Grandma pointed out the star and told us this story.

Once upon a time in Greece a beautiful boy was born with shiny black curls like a deep night; creamy, velvety soft skin; and huge blue eyes like two big lakes. His parents named him Ampel. His father was Satyr, one of the lower gods in the Olympus.

Ampel was a creature with a human torso and horse legs, and he was one of the closest friends and companions of the powerful god of wine and merrymaking, Dionysus. His mother was a wood nymph who lived bound up with a tree in the forest. She was a good friend of Ampelos (grapevine) and gave her newborn son the name Ampel in honor and admiration of her.

Ampel grew up surrounded by Satyrs that had horse and goat legs. He went with them everywhere they traveled. He played games with his mother's friends, nymphs which were secondary goddesses embodying the forces of Nature. The forest's nymphs, called dryads or wood nymphs, like his mother, told him mysterious stories about the forest and its green inhabitants. The naiads, the nymphs of lakes and rivers, taught him how to swim and told him stories about how they derived their vitality from, and in turn gave up their lives to, the water in which they dwelled.

Once when Ampel was playing in the forest with his dryad friends, he saw burgundy grapes hanging from the crown of an elm tree. The grapes looked so attractive, beautiful, and juicy that he wanted to pick and eat them. He climbed the tree and tried to tear off a branch of grapes, but he could not keep his balance and he fell to his death.

When the nymphs found him, they told the god Dionysus in desperation about the young man. Dionysus loved him like he was his own son. He was very upset when he saw Ampel lying dead in the grass, wounded and breathless, but he was powerless to bring him back to life.

"I will not give him to Hades, the god of the Underworld, who will take him into his dark Kingdom of the Shadows, the gloomy subterranean land of the dead. I will place his soul in the sky among the stars." And he did so before Capon, Hades' servant, could transport Ampel's soul through Styx, the underground river of Hate, which led to the Kingdom of Shadows.

Ampel had been transformed by Dionysus into a magnificent bright star, Vindemiatrix, the so-called "grape star." Every night it shines in the sky with all seven colors of the rainbow.

"You see now it shines above all vineyards on earth— like no other in the sky," explained Grandma, "and you will always find it without mistake."

My sister and I looked at the dark night sky with the big luminescent, multicolored star shining above and wondered if it could see us thinking at this moment about the sad destiny of a young man with the romantic name of Ampel. And Grandma, sensing our question, said, "You know, I believe that he is like a guiding light to many good things that happen to people on the earth."

One of these good things is a treatment with grapes, a new and effective direction in alternative medicine which was recently introduced. I call this method *ampelotherapy*. It is widely used in well-known health resorts in Russia and Ukraine—wellness centers in the Crimea and Caucasus Mountains region. There is much evidence that *ampelotherapy* is used as a natural treatment because of its strong curative powers and its ability to produce good results in many cases especially for people with nervous tension, tiredness, a weakened immune system, involuntary weight loss, or heart and respiratory disorders, and patients in a stage of recovering after some serious surgeries. People are rejuvenated as proof that this unique system works because *ampelotherapy* is a combination of pure natural ingredients given to people by the generous goddess of Earth. These are grape berries, fresh grape juice, tasty mineral water from a local spring, clean air full of oxygen, thousands of evergreens and beautiful flowers, and basking almost all year around in a pleasant environment which is not affected at all by pollution, humidity, or urbanism.

As you see, the explanation of this success is simple. It is a treatment with juicy grapes, combined with the refreshing, clean, and aromatic air quality in the warm, continental climate.

Warning:

Despite having great medicinal properties, grapes can provoke aftereffects and acute conditions of the stomach and heart, ulcers, breath shortage accompanied by swelling and hypertension, and intestinal pains. The overuse of grapes can promote obesity. Those who suffer from chronic disease of the lungs or have dental problems should consult a health-care practitioner before undertaking grape therapy.

The following can lower high cholesterol:

 34. Drink ½ cup fresh grape juice three times a day one hour before a meal. Start with ½ cup and do it for one month. During the fifth week take one cup three times a day one hour before meals. During the sixth week take two cups three times a day one hour before meals. The complete treatment is recommended for six weeks.

Grapes contain sugar-glucose and fructose, which are easily absorbed by the body. It is very useful in a treatment of many diseases.

Your physician or health-care practitioner should determine your treatment with *ampelotherapy*, based on your medical history. Russian and

Ukrainian physicians usually prescribe *ampelotherapy* for two to six weeks. The length of time is determined by the doctor for each patient individually.

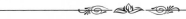

 35. A patient enrolled in *ampelotherapy* treatment eats the bulk of the grapes in the morning 30 minutes before breakfast. The remaining grapes (up to four pounds) are eaten over the course of the day. The grapes should be ripe and thin-skinned for this treatment. See #36.

 36. As a natural healer and preventive, one bunch of grapes could be eaten two to three times a day one hour before meals. This is enough time for the body to absorb all nutritious elements provided by this plant.

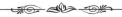

Usually grape treatment begins with a small dosage: 300 grams or about 10 ounces a day and gradually increases to two kilograms or about four pounds. It is recommended to stop eating fatty foods and dairy products, including raw milk, when using this treatment. Kasha or porridge is permissible if it is made from whole grains such as organic steel-cut oatmeal, buckwheat, millet, barley, or roasted wheat cereal and cooked with water. Raisins (1–1½ ounces) or honey (one teaspoon) can be added to these porridges.

> **Warning:**
>
> Don't drink grape juice in large quantities if you are diarrhea sensitive or you have diabetes, obesity, stomach ulcer, or chronic inflammatory processes in the lungs. Consult your physician or health-care practitioner.

Grape therapy is not recommended for people with obesity and serious heart problems, high blood pressure, critical forms of tuberculosis and abscesses, inflammation in the lungs, and other sicknesses in acute stages. Consult your doctor. Don't make independent decisions without consulting a professional health-care specialist.

What kind of grapes are used in *ampelotherapy*? Vitis-Isabella and Muscat are beneficial for chronic bronchitis. Semillon and Riesling heal patients vulnerable to infections in their rehabilitation period from viral and bacterial infections (persistent colds, repeated flu) or those suffering cardiac, vascular, kidney, and liver problems. Tender and juicy Muscat and Silvaner are effective in treating metabolism disorders.

Don't take more than 1 to 1½ quarts of grape juice per day.

Now you know that grapes can treat people with different diseases, but grapes and the juice of this berry of life have also saved thousands of young and healthy soldiers on the battlefield with the help of birds well known to all of us. These birds are snow-white storks.

Precaution:

Do not eat raisins in large quantities (more than two pounds)! They can provoke intestinal disorders.

Long, long ago during the Russian-Turkish war, the Fortress Gorodeshty in Moldova was under siege by the Turks. Thousands of defenders of the fortress courageously fought the enemies. All their reserves of food and fresh water came to an end and they began to lose their energy and couldn't bear the siege anymore. The Russian and Moldavian soldiers were close to death. Their hopes were dashed, and the enemies were already celebrating their victory.

Suddenly a flock of white storks flew in to the hills, where the vines grew under the sun. They took bunches of sun-ripened grapes in their beaks and brought them to the people in the fortress. Dying from starvation and thirst, the soldiers ate these life-giving berries and were immediately refreshed. They became strong and brave with renewed vigor and held the fortress against enemy attacks. The Turkish soldiers were forced to retreat in confusion.

From that time on, people never forgot these special and kind birds that saved their lives and helped them gain victory in such a difficult battle. Some people still believe that a white stork, bearing a bunch of grapes in his beak, will bring them good luck, happiness, and success. Storks also bring newborn babies to couples, as you know.

In the villages of Moldova and in the Ukraine, people call white storks "the sacred birds." These birds are seen on the roofs on many houses in the countryside there. They bustle about people who want to be happy and have children, and they are more than welcome, as the most desirable guests and messengers of good luck and exciting news.

One morning I went with Grandma to our vineyard. A snow-white stork was already a guest there. But he was not really a guest. On the contrary, we were guests. He was walking like a very important "person" in our vineyard. He walked slowly but surely on the tops of the vines. He looked proudly at us and took wing with one stroke. My breath was taken away. This wonderful creature of Nature—this small, courageous, delicate, and kind bird—was so beautiful and amazing!

I just stopped for a minute and looked at him. He was right there, where the blue sky was bottomless, the hills were foggy-blue, and a golden sunrise gave a beginning to a new day full of good luck, a fine mood, and vital energy.

Grandma was looking at the blue expanse of morning sky and said, "It's Ampel who sent this miracle, the stork, to us. Look at the sky. It will remind you that you live in this wonderful world, you are healthy and happy, and you should be always grateful for that."

It always surprised me how my tiny, old, and loving Grandma had an amazing ability, even in sad stories like Ampel, always to see something good and happy. I guess she looked very often to the sky. You may think this a strange thought, but it is not so strange after all. Ancient people said that if you look at the sky for a short time, especially in the morning, it will dispel evil from you. It is as if by meditating on the sky that you cleanse yourself of all negative thoughts and wrong actions.

Dried grapes—raisins—are included as a main ingredient in the treatment of seriously ill people and those recovering from surgery. They help them to overcome weakness and fatigue and gain renewed energy, which they lost fighting the disease. Raisins help also those feeling down or exhausted due to changes in weather conditions.

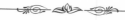

 37. Mix seven ounces each of raisins, dried apricots, and dried prunes. Chop in a food processor. Chop 25–30 small walnuts and mix them well with the dried fruit. Your natural medicine is ready to eat. Put it into a glass jar with a tight-fitting lid and keep in the refrigerator. Take one full tablespoon a day and drink eight ounces low-fat buttermilk or kefir. This mixture strengthens your immune system to sustain any infections and brings a good supply of energy. You can give one full teaspoon of this mixture to your child recovering from a cold or flu, along with ½ cup of low-fat buttermilk or kefir.

High-calorie raisins are a good, nutritious product and are very effective as a diuretic, to eliminate gall-stones, to enrich the blood, and to rejuvenate your body. Raisins are especially good for people suffering from arrhythmia and heart weakness.

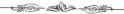

 38. Make ½ cup strong Indian, Ceylon, or Earl Grey black tea. Add one teaspoon honey. Mix well and pour ½ cup fresh grape juice into the tea. One cup of this tea-grape juice drink is a good natural healer for such difficult conditions as intestinal or stomach disorders and dysentery.

39. If you suffer from bronchitis or bronchial asthma, go in June to the Napa Valley in California or another vineyard. Walk there for at least one hour and breathe in the smell of small, delicate green flowers of the blossoming grapevines. Eat one cluster of green table seedless grapes a day and you'll feel better. My favorite is so-called "Lady's Fingers" because the berries have an elongated, oval form like long, graceful women's fingers.

In our supermarkets I have found good brands from organic vineyards suppliers.

You can also drink one glass of white natural grape juice.

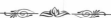

40. Gather fresh grape leaves. Wash them well and dry outdoors under the sun. Then beat or mill the leaves in a mortar to make a powder. Take one to two teaspoons with one cup warm water to stop uterine bleeding.

Nastoykas (specially prepared liquors, infusions, and decoctions made with grape leaves, can treat skin disorders, according to Tibetan medicine.

 41. Wash 10–15 grape leaves and put them in a pot with two cups boiling water. Boil for 10 minutes. Then leave to infuse for 15 minutes. Warm up again, if needed. Soak a towel in this infusion and use as a compress or wash irritated skin with it.

 42. Make vegetarian grape *golubtsi* or "grape leaves." This is the most enjoyable way to treat yourself with a nutritious and healthy meal.

43. Make a healthy grape compote or "Rainbow berries," which is also one of our family recipes. Wash two to three bunches black grapes. Put them in a pot with four cups cold spring water. Bring to a boil. Cook 10 minutes. Mix in one tablespoon sugar, honey, or fructose. Put a small bunch of grapes in a tall, wide, clear glass jar and pour grape concoction over it. This nutritious dessert tastes yummy and it looks very attractive with a grape cluster "swimming" inside. Enjoy!

Here is my grandma's recipe:

*P*repare 30–40 young grape leaves; two table-spoons olive oil, corn oil, or butter; two onions; 10–12 baby carrots; one parsley root; ½ cup uncooked rice, two tablespoons tomato puree or three freshly cubed tomatoes; ½ cup lemon juice; ½ cup sour cream; one cup chicken broth; one cup tomato juice, two teaspoons sugar or honey; one teaspoon salt; ½ teaspoon black pepper; one teaspoon fresh dill; and one tablespoon fresh parsley.

Pour boiling water on the grape leaves and wash them well. Blanch the rice by rinsing in a sieve in cold water. Mix and roast a little bit of diced onions, carrots, parsley root, and parsley leaves. Put blanched rice and all roasted vegetables in a big bowl. Add salt and pepper, chopped fresh dill, and parsley leaves. Mix well. Make balls with this vegetable stuffing and put one on each prepared grape leaf. Roll each into a small "package."

Rub the walls and the bottom of a two-quart pot with olive oil. Cover the bottom of the pot with grape leaves. Carefully place the golubtsi layer by layer in the pot. Mix chicken broth with tomato juice or tomato puree and a pinch of salt and black pepper. Mix two tablespoons lemon juice with two teaspoons sugar or honey and pour this liquid into the pot. Cook 10 minutes. Cover the tops of the golubtsi with grape leaves and put pot in a 350° oven and let it steam until the rice is ready (about 25–30 minutes). Place all golubtsi on a big serving plate. Pour the sauce remaining in the pot on top of the golubtsi. Top with dollops of sour cream. Chop fresh parsley and sprinkle on top. Serves 5–10, warm or cold.

This is a delicious and healthy meal. You can add to the vegetable stuffing one pound of ground veal for a nice fla-vor. Then you can enjoy a small bunch of grapes, or one cup grape juice or one cup grape *compote* for dessert (see #43).

Do you know that sometimes even a happy grapevine cries with juicy tears? According to Avicenna, an ancient Asian doctor, the tears of a grapevine heal herpes (shingles). The juice, flowing out when the grapevine is cut, or a juice exuded when the grapevine burns is called a grapevine's tears. Ancient people used it by soaking a cotton pad in grapevine tears and applying to an affected area.

A grapevine was always a symbol of friendship and constant affection for the family and friends—especially for Russians. Century after century many different enemies invaded this grape country. Moldova is located in the southeastern part of Europe on the major European crossroads. The climate is moderate and the soil is rich and black, similar to the famous fruitful soil in Switzerland, Italy, and France. Hundreds of vineyards grow there under the friendly rays of the sun and blossom with a fancy appearance in the long valleys. Thousands of liters of red, white, and rosé wines and juices are made every fall.

Even on a topographical world map, the contours of this country resemble a bunch of grapes. For many centuries it attracted numerous invaders: Scythians, Hottentots, Huns, Golden Horde of Tatars and Mongolians, ancient Romans, and Turks. Wars raged on and on beginning in the twelfth century.

My grandfather's family lived in Moldova for centuries, learning how to be happy and how to keep a healthy spirit in a healthy body.

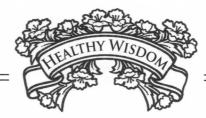

The sun, with all those planets revolving around it and dependent on it, can still ripen a bunch of grapes as if it had nothing else in the universe to do.

—*Galilée (Galileo Galilei), 1564–1842, Italian physicist and astronomer*

Life well spent is long.

—*Leonardo Da Vinci (1452–1519), Florentine artist and scientist*

*Throw nature out of the door, it will come back (or return)
through the window.*

—Fyodor Dostoevsky (1821–1881), Russian novelist, The Brothers Karamazov

If you want the present to be different from the past, study the past.

—Baruch Spinoza (1632–1677), Dutch philosopher

First say to yourself what you would be; and then do what you have to do.

—Epictetus (C.A.D. 55–135), Greek Stoic philosopher

The heart has its reasons which reason knows nothing of.

—Blaise Pascal (1623–1662), French scientist and religious philosopher

*I know of no more encouraging fact than the
unquestionable ability of man to elevate his life
by a conscious endeavor.*

—Henry David Thoreau (1817–1862), American writer

If you want to be happy, be...

—Alexei Tolstoi (1883–1945), Russian novelist and playwright

A likely impossibility is always preferable to a convincing possibility.

—Aristotle (384–322 B.C.), Greek philosopher

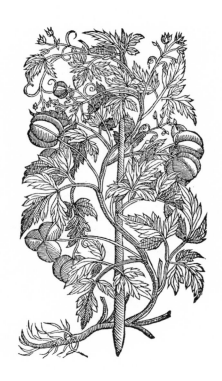

Chapter 4

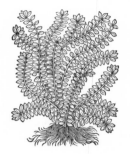

Stop Sneezes and Sniffles
and Stifle a Cold

Nature teaches beasts to know their friends.

—*William Shakespeare (1564-1616), English playwright and poet*

FACTS

According to some estimates, people in the United States suffer one billion colds annually. Children have about 6 to 8 colds a year. In families with children in school, the number of colds per child can be as high as 12 a year. Adults average 2 to 4 colds a year although the range varies. Women, especially those aged 20–30 years, have more colds than men, possibly because of their closer contact with children.

More than 200 different viruses are known to cause the symptoms of the common cold, reports the American Lung Association.[14] In addition, the National Center for Health Statistics (NCHS) Report shows that 7 in 10 adults are not active regularly. Is it any surprise then that physician visits reached 824 million in 2000?

Let your vital power work for you. When you get a cold, see it as a red flag that your body has accumulated too many toxins and lost its internal purity. Let a stuffy nose be a sign that it is time to take the "trash" out and to relax and nurture yourself.

Twelve Months

*O*nce in a small village in Russia lived Mariushka, a delightful young girl. After her mother died, her father married an evil woman. The woman did not love her new stepdaughter, Mariushka, and forced her to be a slave to her and to her daughter.

On a frosty January day, icy trees stood amidst other snowy shapes. Animals hid in their dens, not daring to show their noses outside. Meanwhile a wicked and jealous woman thought of tedious tasks meant to tire Mariushka so she would lose her freshness and not be more beautiful than her lackluster daughter.

The old woman ordered Mariushka to go into the forest and pick snowdrops for her daughter's birthday the next day. Mariushka reminded her that snowdrops bloom in March not January. The stepmother persisted, "Go to the forest and find these flowers under the ground. If you do not find them, do not come home."

Mariushka went crying into the bitterly cold forest where the strong northern wind blew and a snowstorm ensued. Mariushka trudged into a clearing where 12 young and old men stood royally dressed in rich blue and gold clothing. They were surprised to see the tiny girl, dressed shabbily in a thin coat full of holes. Mariushka told them her sad story.

The men were filled with compassion. The oldest man struck the ground with his cane and cast a spell. At once the coldest month of January ran away. The second man did the same, and February disappeared instantly. The third man raised his cane and warmth spread throughout the air; the sun appeared and the gray sky turned bright blue. As each man took his turn, each month's passing hastened the seasons along.

Milky, tender flowers bloomed throughout the meadow. The 12 men smiled and said, "Take as much as you can carry home. We did for you what we could, and we hope that your stepmother will be happy now."

The poor girl, laden with snowdrops, ran back to her stepmother, sure that the vile-mannered woman would be amazed by her accomplishment. However, the stepmother appeared unimpressed, and Mariushka, suffering from a cold she had caught in the woods, was left alone to nurse herself back to health.

Fortunately she understood the powers of healing herbs and became well overnight. Amazed that Mariushka had recovered so quickly, her stepmother begged her to teach her about herbs and stopped placing impossible demands upon her.

Nature knows best how to rid the body of toxins

When you get a cold, Mother Nature will help you cleanse and purify your body. Allow your body's defenses to restore it to health. Do not disturb the process. Whenever my sister and I were young and caught a cold, Mama prescribed fasting. And, of course, we were to adhere to the following rules:

 1. Put yourself (or your children) in a warm bed.

 2. Go without food, including fruits and fruit juices.

 3. Drink distilled water with honey and lemon and herbal teas.

 4. Keep your bedroom refreshed and inviting.

 5. Refrain from reading, watching TV, or listening to the radio.

 6. Keep talking to a minimum.

 7. Sleep as much as you can and relax during this cleansing process.

I call treating a cold "cleaning house." Treatment usually lasts from one week to 10 days, regardless of the medicine you take. By following the simple methods that I mentioned above, it sometimes took my sister and me only three days to recover. Those days of relaxation and isolation restored our health and happiness (as Bernard Shaw said in *Back to Methuselah*, "I enjoy convalescence. It is what makes the illness worthwhile.") Most importantly we did not put any over-the-counter drugs into our body.

I used these simple remedies with my sons when we lived in southeastern Europe. The weather, with the exception of summer, was cold, windy, rainy, and snowy. My oldest son was a member of a professional water polo team. He began playing when he was in first grade and played year-round in an outdoor pool with heated water. Water polo players often suffer from nose and ear ailments and my son was no exception. He would get a stuffy nose and otitis–ear infections. I used the magic phrase, "Go without food" with him many times. Fasting always helped to hasten his recovery.

Try the following infusions to rid the body of toxins.

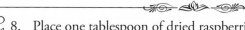

8. Place one tablespoon of dried raspberries in eight ounces of boiling water. Steep for 20 minutes. Filter and drink one cup of hot raspberry tea twice daily—once before you go to bed.

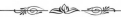

9. Combine one teaspoon dried raspberries and one teaspoon peppermint flowers with one cup boiling water in a glass jar. Cover with a lid and steep for 20 minutes. Filter and drink one cup of hot tea before bedtime as a diaphoretic medicine.

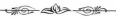

10. This folk recipe originally called for coltsfoot herb, which has been used at least for 2,500 years as an effective demulcent and expectorant. Coltsfoot contains pyrrolizidine alkaloids, which may be toxic to the liver, but these alkaloids are largely destroyed when boiled to make a concoction.

Combine two teaspoons raspberries, one teaspoon marshmallow root, and one teaspoon wild marjoram. To one tablespoon of the mixture, add one cup boiling water. Steep for 20 minutes, filter, and drink ½ cup of the hot drink three or four times a day as a diaphoretic.

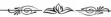

11. Make an herbal composition of one teaspoon dried raspberries, two teaspoons raspberry leaves, two teaspoons wild marjoram, and two teaspoons marshmallow root. Add 10 ounces boiling water to one tablespoon of the herb mixture. Boil slowly 5-10 minutes in an enamel pot, filter, and drink ½ cup of hot tea three to four times a day before a meal as a diaphoretic and expectorant.

Pregnant or nursing women or children under six should not use coltsfoot.

We have substituted marshmallow (Althea officinalis) to replace it in this recipe and other recipes that list a demulcent.

 12. Make our family cream "Magician" No.1. This is a simple and effective folk remedy to alleviate coughs and clear lung congestion. Combine two teaspoons butter with one teaspoon flour or starch and two teaspoons honey (not tropical). Mix until thickened and take one teaspoon three to four times a day along with hot chamomile tea and lemon for one to two weeks.

 13. Combine one tablespoon linden flowers and one tablespoon rose hips with one cup boiling water and boil five minutes. Filter and drink one cup before bedtime. This infusion is soothing for colds and flu, and it is a good treatment for rheumatism.

 14. Two tablespoons raspberries
One tablespoon wild marjoram
Use the same method as in #13.

 15. Combine in an enamel pot one teaspoon dried leaves of peppermint and one teaspoon black elder flowers in one pint boiling water. Boil 5–10 minutes, filter, and drink one to two cups before bedtime.

 16. Combine one tablespoon linden dried flowers and one tablespoon black elder flowers with one cup boiling water in a pot. Strain and drink before bed.

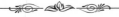

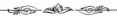

17. Red bilberries are popular in people's medicine. This "mountain cranberry" is effective as a juice or tea to treat colds. Combine one tablespoon fresh red bilberries in a pot with one cup water. Boil, add honey, and drink one hot cup two to three times a day.

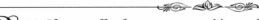

18. If you suffer from a severe cold, try this remedy. Combine one small twig of red bilberry with one cup of boiling water in a glass jar. Steep for 30 minutes, filter, and take two tablespoons four to five times a day.

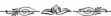

19. Eat two to three pieces of garlic every day as a preventative measure during flu season.

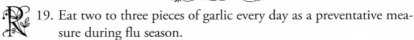

20. Combine one tablespoon dried Siberian elder flowers with one cup boiling water. Steep for 20 minutes, filter, and drink 2½ ounces three to four times a day 15 minutes before eating. Sweeten with honey if desired.

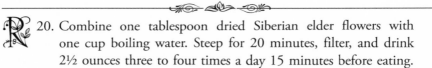

21. Make birch vodka or birch tincture. To one pint of vodka, add ¼ ounce of dried birch buds in a glass jar. Steep for two weeks in a cool place. Filter and take 15-20 drops to one teaspoon, dissolved in boiling water, before a meal. This assists in treating a cold, flu, inflammation of the kidney and liver, skin diseases, and rheumatism.

22. Combine one teaspoon each of elder flowers, linden flowers, chamomile, willow bark, blackthorn flowers, and mullein flowers with one cup of boiling water. Steep 15 minutes, filter, and drink two to three cups a day.

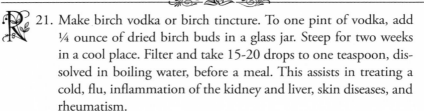

23. Mix one teaspoon each elder flowers, chamomile flowers, linden flowers, and mint leaves. To one tablespoon of the mixture, add one cup of boiling water. Steep for 20 minutes, filter, and drink ½ cup of the hot drink three to four times a day as a diaphoretic.

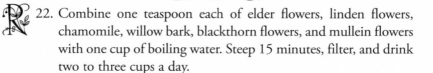

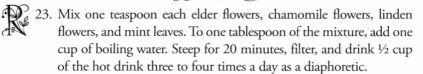

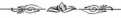

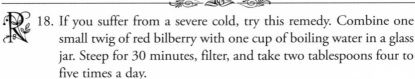

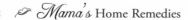

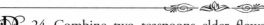

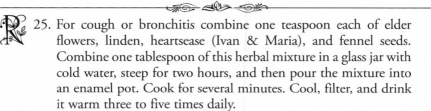

24. Combine two teaspoons elder flowers, two teaspoons linden flowers, two teaspoons willow bark, one teaspoon licorice root, one teaspoon chamomile flowers, and one teaspoon poppy petals. Combine two tablespoons of this herbal composition in a large glass with one pint of boiling water. Cover, steep for 15 minutes, then filter and drink warm during the day.

25. For cough or bronchitis combine one teaspoon each of elder flowers, linden, heartsease (Ivan & Maria), and fennel seeds. Combine one tablespoon of this herbal mixture in a glass jar with cold water, steep for two hours, and then pour the mixture into an enamel pot. Cook for several minutes. Cool, filter, and drink it warm three to five times daily.

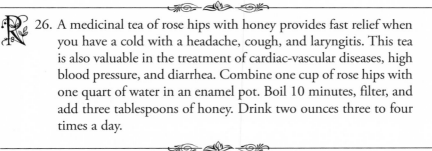

26. A medicinal tea of rose hips with honey provides fast relief when you have a cold with a headache, cough, and laryngitis. This tea is also valuable in the treatment of cardiac-vascular diseases, high blood pressure, and diarrhea. Combine one cup of rose hips with one quart of water in an enamel pot. Boil 10 minutes, filter, and add three tablespoons of honey. Drink two ounces three to four times a day.

Hot teas, cold compresses, and warm hearts keep colds at bay

27. Pour ½ cup of olive or sunflower oil in a glass jar and add one tablespoon of minced marsh cudweed (*Gnaphalium uliginosum*) leaves. Shake daily while allowing to steep for 21 days. After three weeks wring out and filter. On the first day of treatment, use two to three drops of this natural medicine in each nostril. Then on each successive day for one week, pour only one drop in each nostril three to four times a day. This medicine can be kept in the refrigerator two to three weeks. It is anti-inflammatory and tones up the respiratory system.

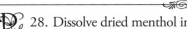

28. Dissolve dried menthol in a pot with boiling water. Tent your head with a towel and breathe in the vapors from above the pot.

29. Dot menthol oil on your forehead, face, and nose and behind the ears.

30. Combine one tablespoon chamomile, two tablespoons licorice root, two tablespoons thyme, and two tablespoons marshmallow flower. Take two ounces three to five times daily after a meal. This is a natural cough suppressant.

31. Juice fresh beets. Use five to six drops in each nostril three times a day.

32. Mix two parts fresh beet juice with one part honey. Insert three to four drops in each nostril three times a day.

33. Combine one tablespoon fennel seeds, two tablespoons marshmallow root, and two tablespoons licorice root. Put one teaspoon of the herb mixture in a mug and add boiling water. Steep for 20–30 minutes, filter, and take one tablespoon a day.

Warm baths can be soothing and relaxing in cold and flu treatment. Try some of these fragrant, mixed herbal baths.

34. Chamomile and linden bath. Combine two ounces each chamomile flowers and linden flowers with one quart water in an enamel pot. Boil slowly for 15–20 minutes. It is a fever-reducing treatment and also helps sleeplessness or skin irritation.

35. Salty bath. Dissolve two pounds of sea salt or iodized salt in a warm bath. This bath cleans, tones the skin, strengthens muscles, and restores the body.

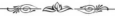

 36. Place one teaspoon of young branches and twigs of white oak bark (*Quercus alba*) or English oak bark (*Quercus robur*) in a two-quart pot. Add about one quart of cold water. Let steep for two hours, then bring to a boil and boil for 30 minutes. Filter this decoction and pour all into bathtub. This remedy acts as an antiseptic and fever-reducer in healing colds. It is helpful in treating tonsillitis, laryngitis, mouth and throat inflammation, bacterial and viral infections if you prepare a fresh decoction daily by boiling four teaspoons of oak per one quart of water for 10–15 minutes. Strain the liquid and gargle. Don't use these preparations for more than two to three weeks. Thanks to the rich content of astringent substances called tannins, the 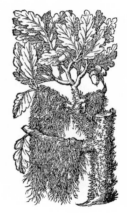 same oak bark liquid can be used in compresses, applied loosely to the affected area until the moisture evaporates, in such cases as weeping eczema and other skin rashes and in healing wounds.

 37. After taking a bath, prepare one cup warm water with one tablespoon honey and drink before bedtime. This natural sedative promotes sound sleep and regulates stomach activity.

 38. Nettle tincture. Combine two tablespoons of nettle with one pint of vodka in a glass jar. Cover with a lid and wrap with cheesecloth. Keep the jar on a window sill for the first day. Store for the next eight days in a cool, dark place. Then filter, wring out, and store in a brown glass bottle or jar. Take one teaspoon of nettle tincture on an empty stomach 30 minutes before breakfast and one teaspoon before bedtime. Continue to take all of this tincture.

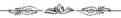

One Hundred Brains

A crane flew up to the Altai as soon as the sun was hot in the spring. He began to dance because he felt so happy to be back in his favorite and familiar marsh. He moved his feet up and down. He lowered and then lifted his wings. He turned his head round and round and bent his neck.

A hungry fox ran by. She was envious that the crane looked so healthy and happy, and she yelped, "I look at you and do not believe my eyes. You dance, poor crane, but you have only two feet."

The crane stopped dancing, looked at the fox, and saw that she had four paws!

"Oh! There is not one tooth in such a long beak!" the fox continued. She smiled and revealed a mouth full of teeth. The crane closed his beak and hung his head. The fox continued to taunt him.

"Where have you hidden your ears and what do you have inside of your head?"

"I found my way here from oversees," the crane almost cried. "That shows that I have some small brain in my head."

"You are so unfortunate," said the fox. "Two feet, but only one brain. Look at me: four feet, two ears, a mouth full of teeth, one hundred brains, and a remarkable brush (tail)."

The crane stretched his neck and saw a man far away with a bow on his shoulder and a quiver of arrows at his belt.

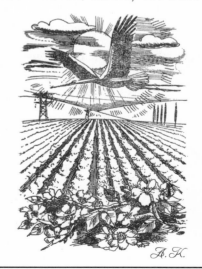

"Your Honorable Fox, you have four feet, two ears, and a marvelous brush. Your mouth is full of teeth and you even have one hundred brains instead of one. But look! A hunter is coming. How can we save ourselves?"

"Well, my one hundred brains give me one hundred suggestions. I don't know which one to follow," the fox cried.

She then plunged into a badger's hole and the crane followed her. The hunter never in his life had seen a crane and a fox living peacefully together. He put his hand inside the hole and pulled the crane out. The crane's legs hung loosely from his body. His eyes were glazed over and his heart nearly stopped beating.

"He obviously had little air to breathe in the hole," said the hunter as he tossed the crane to the ground. In the meantime the fox grew impatient and curious as to what was going on. She ran out of the hole and right into the hunter's bag!

"Perhaps I will put the crane in my bag too," the hunter thought. "It can be a good meal for my dogs."

But the crane had taken flight and was flying so high that even an arrow would not reach him. The fox, who had a hundred brains, a mouth full of teeth, two ears, and a remarkable brush, had been caught, but the crane who thought logically with only one brain had made the right choice and saved himself.

We can use herbal remedies in beneficial ways without having "one hundred brains." They are easy to make; they are natural and do not have complicated side effects as many chemical drugs do.

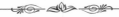

39. Create onion drops. Grate a small onion to make a fresh juice and add the same quantity of water. Use a medicine dropper to insert two to three drops in each nostril. In one to two days these drops will treat inflamed nasal membranes; stuffy, runny nose following a cold; and sinus pain. It will also soften a cough, which often occurs with infections such as colds or influenza.

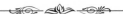

 40. Try the following two simple exercises: To treat a headache, with your fingers massage in a circular, clockwise direction your frontal (forehead) sinuses 7–10 times, then massage your nose 7–10 times to help clear nasal congestion.

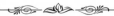

 41. Two quick headache remedies:

a) Take thyme out for tea. Infuse two tablespoons thyme leaves in eight ounces water. Steep 10 minutes, strain, and drink twice a day.

b) Chop one tablespoon feverfew and put into one ounce butter. Spread on bread and eat.

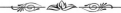

Make a special concoction called "Dog Rose," named after the main ingredient, which the ancient Greeks believed was the best medicine to treat the bite from a dog. This plant is the rose hips (*Rosa canina*), which means dog rose.

For centuries it has been known for its valuable preventive characteristics. Hippocrates, Greek physician and father of medicine, used rose hips berries as natural medicine. Three centuries ago in Russia rose hips were appraised higher in price than gold and were recognized as a rare and important natural medicine.

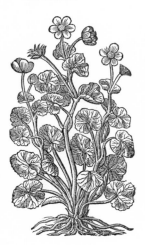

People could get these berries only in exchange for sable fur, velvet, satin, or gold. Rose hips berries were kept in the Kremlin's pharmaceutical stock and the Russian tsar's permission was required to acquire this miraculous healer.

In ancient Russian hand-written encyclopedias of folk medicine is information on rose hips and its effectiveness as a tonic to make gums stronger; to treat cold, flu, laryngitis, gastric diseases, inflammation of the kidneys, liver and bladder problems, anemia, and tuberculosis; and to ease the pain of childbirth. Take advantage of this rich source of vitamin C that Mother Nature generously bestows upon us.

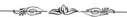

 42. "Dog Rose." Wash two tablespoons dried rose hips in cold water and grind. Combine them with two pints water and, if desired, four tablespoons sugar or honey. Boil for 10 minutes in a covered pot and then steep for two to three hours and filter. Drink one cup in the morning and one cup in the evening. This is a beneficial vitamin drink for children too. If your rose hips drink is unsweetened, limit your intake of the beverage to only two to four ounces a day to prevent an elevated level of stomach acidity.

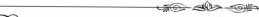

 43. Wash whole rose hips berries and place them in an enamel pot with 16 ounces boiling water and two tablespoons sugar. Boil covered for 10 minutes. Steep for 24 hours and filter. Drink this homemade vitamin medicine as you would juice. During convalescence after illness, it is effective in restoring normal functioning to the stomach and reducing cramping. The old texts assert that it assists "to render harmless" gases and helps to dissolve stones in the bladder and kidneys.

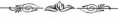

44. Boil two tablespoons of rose hips roots in one cup of water for 15 minutes. Steep until cool and add one teaspoon of honey. Drink ½ cup three times a day for 7–10 days. Increase the quantity by following these ratios:

a) two tablespoons rose hips to one cup water to one teaspoon honey

b) four tablespoons rose hips to 16 ounces water to two teaspoons honey

c) six tablespoons rose hips to 24 ounces water to three teaspoons honey

 45. Rose hips liqueur with vodka. Prepare one cup of dried or fresh rose hips. If you use fresh berries, do not cut them. If you use dried, dice them and combine with 8–12 cups of sugar. Add 24 ounces of vodka and steep in the sun for five days. On the sixth day add 10–24 additional ounces of vodka. Allow mixture

to continue to steep in the sun for five more days. Filter on the 10th day, and take one tablespoon two to three times a day after a meal.

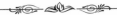

Centuries ago people were inspired by rose hips to write poetic fairy tales and illustrate them with images of beautiful sleeping young women. The arched and curved vines of this plant are closely interwoven and form

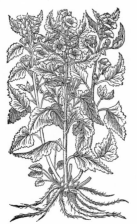

impenetrable brushwoods, which are riddled with sharp, crooked thorns. In Europe this plant blooms in late fall with big, beautiful, and aromatic wild rose blossoms. Because of the dense brush and dangerous thorns, the flowers and tasty berries are inaccessible to wildlife, except birds.

One of the first herbal infusions I became familiar with as a child was marsh cudweed (*Gnaphalium uliginosum*) tea. The herb is a dwarf, evergreen shrub with a strong, camphor-like fragrance.

This herb was well loved by my family, and we had many plants in our stock of herbs to complement it in our home-made infusions or tonics like elecampane; astringents like mullein; elder flowers as a phlegm-reducing herb; or wild lettuce as a cough suppressant. The tea of marsh cudweed is used widely throughout Russia to treat colds, bronchial asthma, and rheumatism. This natural healer is an anti-inflammatory fighter, tones up the respiratory system, and gives temporary relief of persistent, hacking cough and shortness of breath.

Here are several remedies:

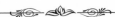

 46. Combine 1½ ounces of marsh cudweed herb in a pot with one quart of boiling water. Steep five minutes and drink about 12 ounces five or six times a day. The course of treatment runs from 5–14 days.

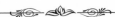

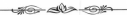

 47. Combine 1/8 ounce marsh cudweed herb and ½ ounce nettle leaves with one quart boiling water and steep five minutes. Drink four ounces five to six times a day. Repeat this procedure for five to seven days.

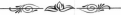

My family used to make another natural medicinal drink called "Bloody tea." It includes another great healing plant, hawthorn (*Crataegus oxyacantha*). This herb's blossoms are sometimes blood red with five delicate petals. The berries of the hawthorn plant are usually red, but sometimes red-yellow. This plant, especially its flowers, is an effective natural medicine for colds.

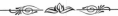

 48. Combine three tablespoons hawthorn flowers with 24 ounces boiling water and steep overnight in a preheated, cooling oven. The next morning filter and warm the mixture. Adults can take one cup three times a day. Children may have two ounces three times a day.

It can be beneficial to eat delicious creams made with black currants because they are rich in vitamin C, glucose, and essential oils. Year-round our herbal stock contained a delicious and effective remedy that we called Black Sofia, which we made from black currants. We named this healing desert Sofia, a woman's name that means wisdom.

49. Make *Black Sofia* vitamin cream. Wash one pound of black currants and dry them on a napkin. Combine with two pounds of organic brown sugar in a blender and whip. Store the mixture in a glass jar in the refrigerator. Drink hot herbal tea, chamomile, linden, mint, raspberry, green tea, or a blend of Indian and Ceylon teas or a glass of warm milk and eat two to three teaspoons of Black Sofia cream. It is a simple remedy, which is also helpful when recovering from colds, tonsillitis, laryngitis, bronchitis, pneumonia, bronchial asthma, headaches, and nervous disorders.

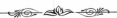

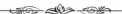

 50. Wash one tablespoon rose hips and combine with 16 ounces boiling water. Boil 10 minutes, cool, filter, and add one tablespoon honey. Mix and drink four ounces three times a day.

 51. To make our family drink, Sweet Kiss, you will need one cup grape juice, 24 ounces spring water, four ounces red wine, (Cabernet Sauvignon), four tablespoons organic sugar or honey, and one grated lemon or orange peel. Bring spring water to the boiling point and add sugar or honey and orange or lemon peel. Boil three to five minutes, cool, filter, and add grape juice and red wine. Pour the liquid from the pot into a glass pitcher. Drink one cup once or twice a day for your recovery and pleasure.

 52. Cherry Milk. Combine one quart of milk with one cup of cherry syrup (carried in supermarkets and health food stores) and one quart of mineral water (S. Pelegrino, Perrier or other). Mix and drink 8–24 ounces a day to cleanse your internal organs.

Natural raspberry and strawberry drinks also help to cleanse internal organs.

 53. Juice 24 ounces of strawberries or raspberries. Add the juice of two lemons, one cup of sugar or honey, and three quarts of mineral water. Mix and drink one cup two or three times a day.

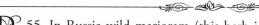

 54. Grandmother's and Grandfather's Old World Sore Throat "Tonic." Sunshine in small doses can be healthy for you. Every day take a seat or lie down on a blanket in the bright sun for five minutes. Face the sun with your eyes closed and your mouth open widely. Sunbeams will penetrate the throat and heal it with its natural warmth and ultraviolet rays. Try this for two weeks.

55. In Russia wild marjoram (this herb is called *dushitsa*) is a one-of-a-kind nectariferous herb which serves as a pungent tonic,

and stimulant. It is a great healer of a sore throat. Combine two tablespoons of wild marjoram with one quart of boiling water. Steep for five to seven minutes. Filter and drink four ounces five to six times daily.

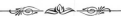

 56. Cow's milk is a great natural healer for people who are not allergic or oversensitive to food irritants. Drink one cup of milk a day.

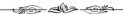

Ivan Pavlov, a world-famous Russian physiologist and experimental psychologist and a Noble Prize laureate in physiology and medicine, said that milk is a product that is perfectly composed by Nature. The health benefits of cow's milk have often been debated in the United States. Many people are lactose intolerant and cannot consume milk in which the lactose has not been removed, but milk has been applauded since ancient times for its healing power. Of course, in ancient times, cows were not given growth hormones and did not eat grass sprayed with pesticides and other chemical "innovations" in powder or liquid form. Fortunately today we can buy organic and lactose-free milk and milk products, which can be used in the many natural medicine recipes throughout this book that list milk as an ingredient.

More than 2,500 years ago in ancient Greece the young son of a rich man became sick with kidney disease. His father sought a healer for his son and invited a well-known physician to his home. This healer's name was Hippocrates. Hippocrates prescribed donkey's milk dissolved in water three times a day for 10 days for this young man.

Ten days passed and Hippocrates then prescribed cow's milk to combat the boy's illness. Following the advice of Hippocrates, the son fully recovered. Hippocrates, who was considered the father of medicine, widely prescribed milk as a treatment for kidney and cardiovascular disease, stress, and stomach problems. He also advised people to drink milk for earaches, anxiety, headache, or nervous disorders. The ancient Egyptians were certain that sick people who bathed in donkey milk would be energized and better able to fight their illness.

Many years ago in Russia, people with various diseases traveled to Moscow from many cities throughout Europe to seek the medical advice of Fedor

Inozemtsev, a medical doctor who was using a "magical" natural medicine to cure his patients. When they learned what his "miracle" treatment was, they were greatly surprised. Dr. Inozemtsev's magical natural medicine was milk—created by Nature.

Force the flu to fly away

Generally flu begins with a stuffy nose, followed by fever, headache, pain in the legs and back, and a cough. Flu can be dangerous because it can develop into bronchitis or pneumonia. The body's immune system can become weak at this time and if the condition goes undetected and is not treated properly, it can provoke nephritis (kidney inflammation) or negatively affect the liver.

Remember: For faster recovery from the flu and nasal congestion:

 57. Take 1,000 mg of vitamin C to block additional infection.

 58. Take a laxative and induce perspiration. Combine three teaspoons each of leaves of linden, mint, and raspberry in a glass jar with two cups of boiling water and steep for 10 minutes. Sweeten with honey. Drink this strong herbal tea and go to bed, covering yourself with a heavy blanket. You will be bathed in sweat, so stay warm and allow the toxins to be released through your pores via your perspiration.

 59. Use a chamomile enema, made with one teaspoon of chamomile to one cup water, once a day for two to three days to flush toxins from the body. Be sure to drink at least eight eight-ounce glasses of water during the day.

 60. Begin a three- to six-day fast, during which you drink chamomile and rose hips teas throughout the day. When you break the fast, maintain a diet of fruits, vegetables, and juice for the next three to four days, making sure that you eat plenty of carrots.

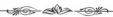

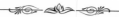

61. Grate a medium-size onion and mix with one pint of scalded milk. Steep 20 minutes in a warm place. Take "Onion Milk" hot before bed. If you cannot drink the whole pint of this medicinal drink, take half in the evening and the second half in the morning. Keep it refrigerated and heat before use the next day.

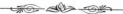

"Onion! Any disease is treated in your arms,'" says an Asian proverb. A Russian proverb salutes the vegetable with "Onion is a healer of seven diseases."

In the Middle Ages doctors already had a strong opinion that even the smell of an onion can help prevent any disease. This is true because an onion contains volatile substances: a high percent of phytoncides acts ruinously against putrefactive pathogenic microbes. Do you know that it is enough to chew a piece of an onion for three minutes and all bacteria will be killed in the mouth? As a first aid remedy, onion is effective in many different health problems. For example, if you cut a fresh slice of onion and put it on insect stings or you apply it on the area affected by nettle rash caused by food allergies, you will get fast relief. The onion is rich with vitamins C, B, and PP and in carotene, glucose, protein, and essential oils.

Hard-working Egyptian farmers cultivated onions, but priests declared the onion a sacred plant and did not use it for food because the modest onion was a symbol of the moon and eternity. The lower classes, however, revered the onion as a wonderful addition to their food. It was recognized as a remarkable stimulant for increasing efficiency and energy.

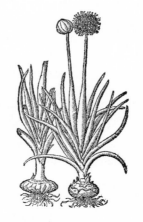

Four thousand years ago construction workers who built the largest pyramid in Egypt, known as the Cheops pyramid, were given onions to eat every day by order of the Pharaoh. It is said that when an ancient Egyptian man had an argument or litigation, he would put in front of him several onions and swear a solemn oath. Grief, despair, and the title of "perjurer" awaited the ignorant man who ate the onion he swore on.

In ancient Greece a beautifully shaped onion was considered a gift to the gods. Roman soldiers were obliged to eat onions every day to enhance their strength and bravery. Scientists in ancient times would cut the onion in two halves to illustrate to their students the structure of the universe, as it was told in the old world, of several spheres surrounding the earth.

In the Middle Ages it was believed that the onion had miraculous powers as a shield from arrows and swords and to ward off the plague. Knights wore an onion on their chests under the armor as a talisman. The onion's flower, attached to the knight's helmet, stood as a symbol to his rivals of defiance to the last breath.

I hope you will be successful in using the sacred onion to help fight diseases and infections. It is sure to bring you increased energy for continued healing. As you know, if you have flu, a cough will likely follow eventually. Get rough with the cough and choke it away! Here's how.

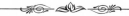

 62. Make organic chicken broth and cook an onion in it. When the onion is tender, eat it at once. Add a pinch of salt for better taste. This cooked onion works magic in treating a cough. Repeat for three to five days.

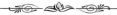

Our family always lovingly teased my grandfather who used this simple folk remedy whenever he had a cough. But guess what? He was always successful in ridding himself of the cough. He strongly believed that the onion would always stop a cough and would even prolong life.

A virus of flu or colds gets into the human body through the respiratory system, takes root in the mucous membranes, and propagates itself very fast. The incubation period is from several hours to several days.

The first symptom we usually see during the first few hours is intoxication with a strong headache, fever, and rheumatic pain throughout the body. Flu/colds often develop complications, such as bronchitis, inflammation of the sinuses, otitis, and pneumonia.

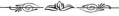

 63. At the onset of symptoms of a flu/cold, take 100 mg vitamin C with a hot green tea and take a hot shower to warm yourself. While taking a shower, massage your chest, face, and neck with a soapy sponge.

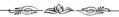

64. If you are sure that your blood vessels and heart are healthy, take a hot bath with chamomile or calendula or add one pint of red wine or apple cider vinegar to the bath water. Go to bed, but after two hours change your pajamas or nightgown. Take a bath or shower every day. The pores of your skin will open, and infection and toxins will be released from your body.

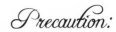

Precaution:

Don't take antibiotics without a doctor's prescription because they don't affect the flu virus. Bacteria in the body get accustomed to antibiotics and these drugs will not then be useful in the treatment of more complicated diseases.

 65. Take two capsules of vitamin C (1,000 mg) in the morning and in the evening, and one capsule of Complex Super vitamin B.

 66. Inhalation therapy. Combine one teaspoon of baking soda with boiling water in a cup. Mix it and breathe in the steam for several minutes.

 67. Combine one tablespoon linden flowers and one tablespoon rose hips with two cups of boiling water and boil 10 minutes. Filter and add several drops of fresh squeezed lemon juice. Drink one to two hot cups of this herbal tea before bedtime.

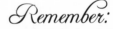

Remember:

Flu/cold virus perishes in an alkaline medium. Baking soda is alkaline.

 68. Combine one tablespoon senna as a laxative, one tablespoon German golden locks, and one tablespoon St. John's Wort. Mix these herbs and bring slowly to a boil in an enamel pot with 24 ounces of water. Boil one minute, filter, and drink three to four times daily, 20 minutes before a meal.

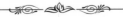

69. Combine one tablespoon buckthorn bark with one tablespoon black elder flowers, which is regarded in folk medicine as a "complete green medical pharmacy." Black elder herb is useful in such conditions as excessive mucus and phlegm. From the seventeenth century it has been one of folk medicine's favorite remedies for "cleansing phlegm," acting as an expectorant, diuretic, and anti-inflammatory and boosting the respiratory system.

70. Make a medicinal drink that our family called Romance, in honor of the Hans Christian Andersen fairy tale, "The Elf of the Rose," written as a romantic story in 1839. Crush dried berries of rose hips. Place three tablespoons rose hips berries and two tablespoons chamomile flowers in an enamel pot with one quart cold water. Boil 10 minutes, cover, and wrap in a thick towel and let steep in a warm place for eight hours. Filter and drink one cup every two to three hours. You may add brown sugar, honey, or jelly to sweeten. If you fast the day that you drink Romance, you will feel much better the next day.

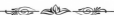

"The Elf of the Rose"

In the midst of a garden grew a rosebush in full blossom. In the prettiest of all the roses lived an elf. He was such a wee thing that no human eye could see him. Behind each leaf of the rose, he had a sleeping chamber.

He was as well formed and as beautiful as a little child could be. He had wings that reached from his shoulders to his feet.

Oh, what sweet fragrance there was in his chambers! And how clean and beautiful were the walls! For they were the blushing eyes of the rose.

During the whole day he enjoyed himself in the warm sunshine, flew from flower to flower, and danced on the wings of the flying butterflies. Then he took it into his head to measure how many steps he would have to take to traverse the roads and crossroads that are on the leaf of a linden tree. What we call the veins on a leaf, he took for roads; ay, and very long roads they were for him; for before he had half finished his task, the sun went down—he had commenced his work too late.

It became very cold, the dew fell, and the wind blew, so the elf thought the best thing he could do would be to return home. He made himself as small as he could, but he found the roses closed and he could not get in. Not a single rose stood open. The poor little elf was very much frightened. He had never before been out at night but had always slumbered secretly behind the warm rose leaves.

Oh, this would certainly be his death. At the other end of the garden he knew there was an arbor, overgrown with beautiful honeysuckles. The blossoms looked like large painted horns, and he thought he would go and sleep in one of these till the morning.

He flew thither . . . but hush! two people were in the arbor—a handsome man and a beautiful lady. They sat side by side and wished that they might never be obliged to part. They loved each other much more than the best child can love its father and mother.

"But we must part," said the young man. "Your brother does not like our engagement, and therefore he sends me so far away on business, over mountains and seas. Farewell, my sweet bride, for so you are to me."

And then they kissed each other, and the girl wept and gave him a rose, but before she did so, she pressed a kiss upon it so fervently that the flower opened.

Then the little elf flew in and leaned his head on the delicate, fragrant walls. Here he could plainly hear them say, "Farewell, farewell," and he felt that the rose had been placed on the young man's breast. Oh, how his heart did beat!

Your heart will beat happily and with great health as you continue your natural treatments.

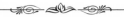

 71. Grate garlic and add one tablespoon of honey. Ratio: 1:1. Take one tablespoon of this medicinal kasha and drink one cup of natural spring water. Mince five tablespoons rose hips berries and combine with one quart cold water in an enamel pot. Bring to boiling and boil 10 minutes. Cover and steep in a warm place, wrapped in a towel for 8–10 hours. Add honey, sugar, or fruit preserves. Drink one cup in the morning and every two to three hours for two days. Gargle with warm water to prevent tooth damage from excess acid.

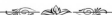

 72. Make the medicinal drink "Trio" as we named it in our family. It includes chamomile, sage, and wood betony. (Wood betony is not commonly used in the United States. It may be hard to track down. Consult the listing of herbal resources in this book.) The root of this herb is bitter and useful in liver treatment with a gentle laxative action. In ancient Europe wood betony (flowers and stems) was used to treat about 30 diseases, including headaches and digestive problems and as a stimulant and cleanser for the system, with a mild diuretic action. In the Middle Ages, this herb was a popular amulet to ward off illnesses or evil. My grandmother knew about it from her old books and used to give it to us when we had colds.

Mince and mix three teaspoons each of chamomile, sage, and wood betony. Combine one tablespoon of the mixture with one pint of boiling water in a glass jar. Cover with a lid, wrap with warm fabric, and let steep for 30–40 minutes. Then filter, add one teaspoon honey, and drink one cup of hot Trio during the day. Also drink one cup of this herbal tea hot before bedtime.

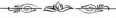

 73. If you have cold or flu together with headache, add peppermint leaves to the herbs in remedy #72. The method of preparation is the same.

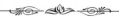

74. If you feel cold as a result of flu, add black elder to the herbal composition: wood betony, chamomile, sage, and peppermint (#72). The method of preparation is the same.

75. Combine equal portions of fresh raspberries, linden flowers, coltsfoot leaves, anise seeds, and willow bark. Combine one tablespoon of the mixture with boiling water, steep covered for 20 minutes, filter, and drink one cup of this tea hot before bedtime as an anti-inflammatory, analgesic, and antiseptic. Use this natural remedy to help reduce fever and relieve a cold's headache and inflammatory conditions.

White willow bark is a valuable ingredient in this remedy. It was used traditionally in people's medicine for fevers. In the nineteenth century many scientists in Europe scientifically investigated this herb, but only one French chemist successfully extracted the active constituent and named it "salicine." This first plant-derived natural "drug" was duplicated later, in 1852, by a chemical in synthetic form as a substance called acetylsalicylic acid. At the end of the nineteenth century it was produced and brought to the world market as aspirin.

One year after this scientific discovery (we wonder if it was coincidence?) Hans Christian Andersen wrote in 1853 a fairy tale, "Under the Willow Tree." See sidebar for an excerpt.

"Under the Willow Tree"

"He was walking one evening through the public roads, the country around him was flatter, with fields and meadows, the air had a frosty feeling. A willow-tree grew by the roadside, everything reminded him of home.

"He felt very tired; so he sat down under the tree, and very soon began to nod, then his eyes closed in sleep. Yet still he seemed conscious that the willow-tree was stretching its branches over him; in his dreaming state the tree appeared like a strong, old man—the "willow father" himself, who had taken his tired son up in his arms to carry him back to the land of home, to the garden of his childhood, on the bleak open shores of Kjoge.

"And then he dreamed that it was really the willow-tree itself from Kjoge, which had traveled out in the world to seek him, and now had found him and carried him back into the little garden on the banks of the streamlet. And there stood Joanna, in all her splendor, with the golden crown on her head, as he had last seen her, to welcome him back.

"And then there appeared before him two remarkable shapes, which looked much more like human beings than when he had seen them in his childhood. They were changed, but he remembered that they were the two gingerbread cakes, the man and the woman, who had shown their best sides to the world and looked so good.

"We thank you," they said to Knud, "for you have loosened our tongues; we have learnt from you that thoughts should be spoken freely, or nothing will come of them; and now something has come of our thoughts, for we are engaged to be married." Then they walked away, hand-in-hand, through the streets of Kjoge, looking very respectable on the best side, which they were quite right to show.

"They turned their steps to the church, and Knud and Joanna followed them walking hand-in-hand; there stood the church, as of old, with its red walls, on which the green ivy grew."

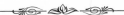

 76. Combine one tablespoon linden flowers and one tablespoon raspberries with two cups water in an enamel pot. Boil five minutes. Steep 10 minutes, filter, and add two tablespoons honey. Drink ½ cup three to four times a day to reduce fever and inflammation.

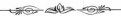

77. Combine one tablespoon elder flowers with one cup boiling water in a glass jar. Place the jar in an enamel pot and steam 15 minutes. Then cool, filter, and add eight ounces boiled water and one tablespoon honey. Take about 2½ ounces two to three times a day as an antiseptic, fever reducer, and expectorant. This can be combined with one tablespoon each peppermint, boneset, and yarrow.

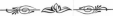

 78. "CCB" natural medicine. For a flu/cold with high fever, place 1⅓ tablespoons chamomile; 1⅓ tablespoons centaury, an Old World herb; and 1⅓ tablespoons bogbean. Add 24 ounces boiling water and steep overnight in a preheated, cooling oven. The next morning filter and warm the healing medicine. Drink three cups a day when the flu is full blown. A cold/flu is a dangerous visitor with bad intentions to destroy our good health, so be patient and well prepared.

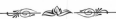

79. "Honey Vodka" is a natural medicine that supports CCB and can be used along with it. Boil 1½ cups vodka with one tablespoon honey. Cool and drink Honey Vodka before bedtime. You might experience sweet dreams and may break into a sweat, which will clear toxins from your body to fight the flu.

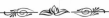

 80. Slice thinly three or four whole lemons and layer in a glass jar. Sprinkle sugar or honey over all. Cover with a lid and eat this natural remedy of vitamin C and glucose four times a day.

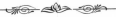

Eat oranges and tangerines or drink natural citrus juices made from organic fruits that you have made fresh in a juicer. Fresh-squeezed juices are best when drunk right away. They contain vitamins A, B, and C and minerals. These natural drinks help us recover faster and improve metabolism. They are known to heal a stuffy, runny nose and prevent the development of atherosclerosis.

The citrus fruits we take for granted in our supermarkets have a varied and interesting background. In the twelfth-century lemons were brought to Italy and Spain from southeastern Africa through the Middle East and northern Africa. Europe first tasted oranges in the beginning of the fifteenth century. It is thought that Vasco de Gamma brought oranges from Palestine to Europe. Even the name orange is in Russian apelsin and came from German apfel, which means Chinese apple (apfe, apple; sin, China). Oranges were cultivated in China 2,200 years before the new era.

The beautiful and tasty southern fruit received high praise in Europe. Europeans began to build special "houses" for growing oranges. These hot houses or green houses are called orangerias in European countries, from the French word orange.

In the beginning of the eighteenth century the glory of the orange shone throughout Russia as well. In 1774 Alexander Menshikov, a fellow of Peter the Great, built a palace named Oranienbaum, which means orange tree in German, with large hot houses to propagate oranges. In 1789 Russian Empress Catherine II ordered that the small town where the palace stood would be named Oranienbaum, complete with its own city emblem displaying an orange tree in a silver field.

Lemons and oranges became popular in Russia as effective natural healers, used widely to treat catarrh of the larynx, to "knit" the bones, to treat rheumatism and scurvy, and to remove toxins from the stomach.

Navigator James Cook brought large quantities of lemon juice to his ships for his sailors during long journeys. In 1795 a special law was mandated that sailors were to have a glass of this medicinal drink every day. The high percentages of vitamins C, A, and B make citrus a real miracle food, an antiseptic healer, and a guardian of our health.

 81. Make a tangerine infusion. Wash three or four tangerines, peel, and dry the skin. Combine the dried tangerine peel with ½ cup cold water in an enamel pot. Bring to a boil and add one tablespoon honey or sugar. Continue to boil for five minutes, then filter and take one tablespoon warm three to four times a day. This soothes symptoms of a cold, flu, bronchitis, or pneumonia.

 82. Combine one cup milk, one tablespoon honey, one teaspoon butter, two eggs, and three to five drops vanilla extract. Boil milk in an enamel pot and cool. Mix honey and butter. Whip eggs, mix in a bowl with honey and butter, and slowly stir in the warm milk and vanilla extract. Drink one cup a day for seven days. It will soothe respiratory problems and cough.

 83. Boil ¾ cup milk and cool. Mix two egg yolks with one tablespoon sugar or honey and while stirring, constantly add the warm milk and three drops vanilla extract. Take this natural medicine for seven days. It provides relief from a cold, nasal rhinitis, sore throat, bronchitis, and pneumonia.

Tangerine Trivia

An Italian merchant from Naples first brought tangerines to Europe. Tangerine in Russian has a musical name, *mandarin*, which came from the Chinese. These fruits were affordable only to the mandarins, the Chinese feudal lords.

You can use all remedies with elder and rose hips when you have a flu.

---

 84. Potato vapors can bring relief. Boil five to six potato skins in a pot with 24 ounces water. When mixture is at a rolling boil, remove from heat and inhale the steam. This simple procedure greatly relieves congestion and improves breathing.

---

 85. To reduce fever, you can use linden flowers alone or in herbal compositions: Combine one teaspoon linden flowers, ½ teaspoon mullein, ½ teaspoon elder with two cups boiling water in a glass jar. Steep for 10 minutes, filter, and drink ½ cup three times a day. You might want to stay home during this treatment because it promotes excessive perspiration.

---

 86. Combine three to four tablespoons of lungwort with one quart of boiling water and steep overnight in a warm place. Reheat in the morning, filter, and take one tablespoon five or six times a day. This herb is soothing and relieves inflammation in the chest.

---

 87. Combine two tablespoons elder flowers with one pint boiling water. The method of preparation is the same as in #85. Drink ½ cup three times a day. Drink hot for feverish and mucous conditions of the lungs or upper respiratory tract.

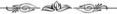

Elder is considered a universal treatment in people's medicine. From the seventeenth century it became a popular remedy to reduce phlegm and encourage perspiration. Ripe elderberries are rich in vitamins, especially A and C, and were used widely in Europe in producing wines and medicinal syrups, which people took as preventive measures against winter colds and respiratory ailments.

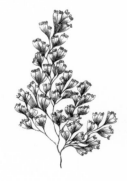

88. Use oat straw medicine as febrifuge (fever reducer). Combine three tablespoons oat straw with one pint boiling water. The method of preparation is the same as in #85. Oat straw is an excellent tonic for the whole system. It is used to treat physical and nervous fatigue and excessive stress. It is ideal for those people with weakened immune systems who suffer persistent colds.

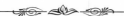

 89. Fill ¼ of a 12-ounce glass jar with Greater celandine and add boiling water to the top of the jar. Steep, cool, filter, and drink ½ cup. This tea can also be used as a gargle. During a flu it can help to restore a normal appetite and sound sleep. It acts as a sedative for the nervous system. Take for seven days 10-15 minutes before a meal and eat with one tablespoon of freshly grated carrots.

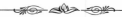

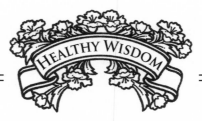

Only with the heart can we see rightly; the essential is invisible to the eye.

—*Antoine de Saint-Exupery (1900–1944), French pilot and poet*

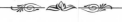

It is not so much our friends' help that helps us as the confident knowledge that they will help us.

—*Epicurus (341–270 B.C.), Greek philosopher*

"Why, one can hear and see the grass growing!" thought Levin,
noticing a wet, slate-colored leaf moving beside a blade of young grass.

—Leo Tolstoy (1828–1910), Russian novelist, from Anna Karenina, 1877

Even if something is left undone, everyone must take time
to sit and watch the leaves turn.

—Elizabeth Lawrence (b.1934), American writer

Cheerfulness is the best promoter of health,
and is as friendly to the mind as to the body.

—Joseph Addison (1672–1719), English writer and statesman

In all things of nature there is something of the marvelous.

—Aristotle (384–322 B.C.), Greek philosopher

[Nature] is the one place where miracles not only happen,
but happen all the time.

—Thomas Wolfe (1900–1938), American novelist

Can you live without a willow tree? Well, no, you can't.
The willow tree is you.

—John Steinbeck (1902–1968), American writer

Everything in nature acts in conformity with law.

—Immanuel Kant (1724–1804), German philosopher

Chapter 5

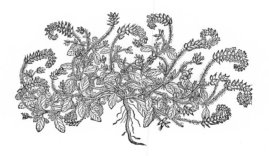

A Sickness of the 21st Century

These people have learned not from books, but in the fields, in the wood, on the riverbank. Their teachers have been the birds themselves, when they sang to them, the sun when it left a glow of crimson behind it at setting, the very trees, and wild herbs."

—Anton Chekhov (1860–1904), Russian playwright and story writer

FACTS

Acccording to the latest information available from the American Lung Association, the Centers for Disease Control and Prevention (CDC), and the National Institute of Allergy and Infectious Diseases (NIAID),

In the United States:

- Allergies affect more than 50 million people.

- Pollen allergy (hay fever or allergic rhinitis) affects nearly 10 percent of the people (26 million people), not including asthma.

- Allergies are the sixth leading cause of chronic disease, costing the health-care system $18 billion annually.

- Chronic sinusitis, most often caused by allergies and the most commonly reported disease, affects approximately 38 million people.

- Allergic drug reactions, commonly caused by antibiotics such as penicillin and cephalosporin, occur in 5 to 10 percent of all adverse drug reactions.

- Eight percent of children six years old or younger experience food allergies. An estimated one to two percent of adults have food allergies.

- A severe allergic reaction known as anaphylaxis occurs in 3.3 percent of the population as a result of insect stings. At least 40 deaths each year result from sting anaphylaxis.[15]

Allergies impact the way millions of people live in America. Here are some more interesting statistics regarding allergies in the United States:

a) Peanut or tree nut allergies affect approximately three million Americans and cause the most severe food-induced allergic reactions.[16]

b) Nine million visits to office-based physicians in 2000 were attributed to allergic rhinitis.[17]

c) Seasonal allergic rhinitis, often referred to as "hay fever," affects more than 35 million people in the U.S.[18]

We are prone to developing allergies when we are under stress or oversensitive. Researchers tell us repeatedly that certain smells, herbs, berries, oranges, and chemicals can provoke allergic reactions and disturb our normal sleep pattern.

Today allergies taunt us and disrupt our daily lives. Many people take allergy medications on a regular basis and, in fact, cannot live a normal life without them.

Austrian doctor Clemens von Piquet coined the term *allergy* in 1906. The first symptoms described by him stated that our body's ability to identify and destroy any harmful organisms such as viruses or bacteria is essential to our survival. People are like most species living on the earth: We have developed our individual immune systems. These systems also target what are considered to be harmless, not dangerous, particles such as flower pollen, dust mite, dust in our homes, or peanuts, causing swelling, inflammation, itching, and, in extreme situations, death.

Today approximately 90 percent of the world population has reactions to various irritants. Why does this happen in 90 percent of people and not in the other 10 percent of the world's population? It happens because 90 percent of people don't realize that their bodies accumulate toxins every day from air they breathe and from the food they eat.

What should we do? The answer is simple. All of us without any exceptions must consistently clean our bodies from these harmful substances poisoning our blood. Like you clean your house at least one time per week, you should clean your body every day using different natural "cleaners." Start your day with a cup of hot water and a piece of lemon before breakfast to "rinse" your blood vessels. Take burdock, 425 mg a day. Make hot peppermint or horsetail tea and add a piece of lemon. Eat baby carrots or drink carrot or birch juice. Enjoy eating melon and salads with grated red beets, almonds, and garlic or cabbage with carrots, apple, and onions. Make your own dressing for salads. It is very easy. Just mix ½ cup of first cold pressed extra virgin olive oil with ½ cup of freshly squeezed lemon juice.

Allergies are so common that even the term *allergy* is frequently used informally in everyday speech. I have overheard people saying to each other, "Oh, leave me alone! Stop it! You talk too much! I have become allergic to you." One day perhaps these statements will be included in a dictionary of colloquial expressions.

When suffering from allergies, try the following unique folk remedy to cleanse your body internally. This method will help you build a strong defense against allergic irritants.

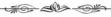

 1. Cleansing Maid, Mama's recipe. Cut two lemons into small cubes. Mince five to six cloves of fresh garlic. Place lemon and garlic into a one-quart jar. Add two tablespoons of honey and fill with boiling water. Let steep until cool and then refrigerate. It will turn a golden amber color with a pleasant taste and lemon aroma. Take one tablespoon three times a day.

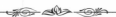

 2. Make horsetail tea. This herb can be purchased in packages in a health-food store. Place one pack of horsetail tea in a cup and add boiling water to fill. Let steep for three to five minutes and drink warm. Drink once every day for 7 to 14 days. Take a two-week break and repeat the treatment.

What is an allergy?

Swiss doctor H. C. A. Vogel wrote in his manual of traditional and complementary medicine that an allergy is a hypersensitivity to a certain kind or variety of different substances. A particular hypersensitivity, he contends, may cause such drastic reactions that it may seem as though the patient has been poisoned.

People with physical hypersensitivity to the environment in which they live are surrounded by allergens—chemical substances; microbes; and the products of their activity, food products, plant pollen, animal proteins, and fats. For instance, some people can become ill if they have ingested only a small amount of egg that is contained in the food they eat. Others eat beans or bread, pastry, or muffins made with wheat flour, or fruit salad with oranges, or any canned food and become critically ill.

Seafood restaurants today are very popular among people who are dieting or concerned with weight gain and cholesterol levels. However I know people who have become ill after eating crabs, lobster, and shellfish while maintaining a normal level of cholesterol. At least their belief that fish contains good cholesterol paid off, and I mean the fish, not shellfish.

Though sad to say, we can count on hundreds of different irritants today that provoke allergic reactions. The following are just some of many:

Industrial: mineral oils, paints, turpentine, nickel, chrome, formalin, urea, and others. Reaction: skin disorders.

Everyday chemicals: lacquers and synthetic colors, detergents and cleansing liquids, cosmetics: soaps, creams, powder, lipstick, eye makeup, hair colorings, shampoos, hair sprays, and nail colors.

Everyday animals: domestic animals (dogs, cats), wool clothing, feathers, usually the dander that penetrates our organism in the form of dust. Chemical and animal irritants usually give us respiratory sicknesses such as catarrh, sinus irritation, cough, rhinitis, and asthma (shortness of breath).

Medical: antibiotics, aspirin (salicylates), various medical drugs, artificial vitamins with preservatives.

Food products: eggs, shellfish, beef, cow's milk, honey, wheat and rye bread, canned foods, citrus fruits (oranges), blueberries, strawberries, nuts, mushrooms, tomatoes, chocolate, artificial colors or flavors, preservatives, chemical solvents, starch, gluten, yeast.

Peanut or tree allergies affect approximately three million Americans a year and cause the most severe food-induced allergic reactions. Any food can turn from a nourishing friend into an allergen/invader. Usually food allergies appear with a break in the order of the normal functions of the stomach/digestive system. Symptoms can include vomiting, diarrhea, and fever.

Floral: flowers, trees, blossoming herbs and grass pollen, essential oils of some plants such as primulas (primrose), tropical plants, hay dust, fungi, daffodils and tiger lilies (which are fragrant in the evening), rhubarb and roses (thorns), and floral smells. Ailments: allergy cold (catarrh, sinus); conjunctivitis; blurry, tearful eyes.

Service machines: home, car and office air conditioners. Although air conditioners provide us with coolness in hot weather, we get processed air instead of the fresh air we need to ventilate our lungs and respiratory system and to supply oxygen to our brain cells. Ailments: allergy cold (catarrh or sinus), sore throat, swollen glands, irritated eyes, common tiredness, head congestion, headache, and asthma.

Natural: sunlight, warmth, hot, or cold could be irritants too, especially in tropical climates. These irritants "sponsor" our body in forming certain substances that become allergens. Ailments: allergy cold, blurry eyes, fatigue, loss of energy, "hot head," headache, skin rash, loss of appetite, and a bitter taste in the mouth.

Street, house, and bookshelf dust: Ailments: asthma and all under Natural.

Smoking: at least 80 different chemicals and metals. Ailments: all of the above.

What factors lead to developing an allergy?

General disorders of normal functions include:

- immune system, which fights an uninvited invader by producing irritation, mucus, and inflammation in our body
- respiratory system
- nervous system
- endocrine system
- circulatory system
- liver dysfunction, a body "sponge," processing blood
- dysfunction of adrenal glands
- traumas of the head and brain
- negative emotions
- irritation
- stress
- smoking
- inappropriate diet
- inappropriate food
- inappropriate life style
- a lack of walking and other exercise
- a shortage of sound sleep

What are allergy ailments?

- allergic arthritis, stiffness in bones, and joint paint; constant urinary infections, cystitis; gynecological problems (yeast infections)
- respiratory: bronchial asthma, asthmatic fit, allergy cold (catarrh, sinus), nasal mucus, sneezing, allergic rhinitis, sore throat
- conjunctivitis (irritated, blurry, tearful eyes)

- hay fever, skin rashes, eczema, blisters
- digestive upsets (diarrhea or constipation), gastric pains
- stress, short-term memory loss, fatigue, loss of energy and appetite

In *The Complete Medicinal Herbal*[19] British author and herbalist Penelope Ody writes, "A healthy system copes with allergens, but if there is tension, infection, or fatigue, the arrival of an allergen tips the balance and an allergic response occurs in the form of hay fever, skin rashes or gastric upsets."

Our immune system is a strong shield, guarding us from uninvited guests—irritants like inflammation, mucus, and phlegm. If we do not treat the symptoms in time, they will continue to penetrate our body and our immune system may become drastically weakened. Allergies are clever invaders. They sometimes hide under a pretty mask that creates a nice image that everything is fine for a while. Then they hit with an ugly, persistent sinus irritation; sore, irritated eyes; urinary infections; arthritic pains; and digestive upsets.

What are common symptoms of allergy?

Allergy symptoms can appear in hundreds of different forms. What to look for?

- "Nettle rash." Blisters and bumps appear on your skin, resembling a burn and maybe the scald of nettle.
- Allergic catarrh (cold). Aspirated human and animal hair or bird feathers (pillows, wool, and mattresses) can result in the swelling of the mucous membranes of the nose and eyes.
- Hay fever or hay catarrh (sinus). Abnormal sensibility to flower pollen, blossoming herbs and trees.
- Under the influence of some irritants, people experience bronchial asthma, shortness of breath, hacking cough, mucous membranes, and bronchial swelling. Red, peeling spots on the skin may indicate eczema. When people suffer from severe eczema, the spots may itch and be wet. Sometimes the spots are withered. Eczema commonly occurs on the hands, feet, and other parts of the body. Types of eczema are different. The condition on the hands is called an irritant contact dermatitis and is caused by everyday contact with substances—irritants

to the skin, such as home chemicals and detergents. The best remedy, doctors say, is to avoid these harmful substances and to keep the skin moisturized. Another type of eczema is a form of allergic contact dermatitis, which usually develops when the body's immune system rebels against some metals, rubber, or certain perfumes coming in contact with the skin. As a matter of fact, many of us wear earrings or belts with buckles made with nickel. Some people experience allergic reactions through repeated contact with this metal or "touch" perfume and develop a skin rash and inflammation. Others between 20 and 40 years of age have so-called infantile seborrheic dermatitis which looks on the scalp like mild dandruff but can be spread to the face, ears, and chest. You may have seen that the skin in this case becomes inflamed or red, then it flakes. Dermatologists believe that yeast growth provokes this condition. What can I say? Many people love to eat sweets. However, consult your doctor, who can prescribe a treatment with antifungal cream. There are two other not very pleasant types of eczema: varicose and discoid. Varicose eczema hits the lower legs of people in their 60s to the late years of their life and is caused by poor blood circulation. To prevent this, walk every day! Move as much as you can and try to prevent this eczema when the skin around the ankles becomes itchy, speckled, and inflamed. If this condition is left untreated, dermatologists say that the skin can break down and an ulcer can follow as a result.

Some people are very surprised and get upset when they see suddenly an appearance of coin-sized red spots on their lower legs and trunk. These "coins" develop fast and become itchy and wet. It is discoid eczema.[20]

As far as I know from my research, there is currently no efficient cure for eczema, but scientists are very optimistic and continue to look for it. However I can assure you that it is possible to find many ways to minimize the distress and discomfort provoked by this condition. The main solution is an effective skin care régime which is easy to conduct. First of all, we can buy many treatments over the counter at the pharmacy, but I would explore the simplest ways to minimize the presence of allergens/invaders in my house. Keep it clean, and keep your body and skin consistently refreshed by taking twice a week a warm bath with 16 ounces of all-natural apple cider vinegar dissolved in it. Keep reading. You'll find further in this chapter more useful natural treatments for eczema tested by folk healers through the centuries. Do not neglect physician consultations and prescriptions. Look to your doctor for professional advice and get a second opinion. It is important to catch a "self-invited invader" at the right time.

What can we do about allergies?

For years, thousands of people have suffered with the ill effects of allergies that have disrupted their daily lives and have been desperate for treatments that would help them regain the normalcy they had before stubborn allergies dictated the way they felt. But until recently medical doctors and world scientists have been stumped for answers.

Currently, I repeat, an estimated 50 million Americans have some form of allergic disease. Approximately 24.7 million people have been diagnosed with asthma, with at least 7.7 million of them children under the age of 18. Asthma is the leading, serious, chronic illness among children in the United States. The good news is that we now can undergo a series of tests to determine specific allergens. Once the allergen is known, a physician can prescribe an effective treatment with well-advertised drugs. No one drug is guaranteed, of course. We are careful about guarantees of any kind.

So what choice do we have? Perhaps we should trust and help ourselves. We are our own best friends and as such we should be educated about our symptoms and the treatment options available to us. For instance, I know that I am very sensitive to antibiotics and food preservatives, strawberries, and the smell of tropical tiger lilies, and I am careful to avoid these irritants. But with allergies you can always expect the unexpected.

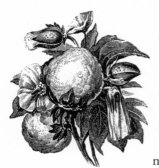

Recently I planted roses in my garden and I pricked several fingers on their thorns. At first I thought that I was not bothered by the cuts at all…until I showered the next morning. It was then that I noticed many red spots on my neck. Curiously they did not itch, and I did not think it was the sign of a serious condition. The next day red spots had spread rapidly over my legs, hands, stomach, and thighs, eventually covering my entire body. In addition to the skin rash, my sinuses became inflamed and I could not breathe normally.

I feared that the rash would spread internally and decided to make an appointment with my physician right away. My advice to anyone who experiences a sudden allergic reaction is to keep a written log of the symptoms before calling your doctor. I recorded the time that the allergic reaction began. Then I listed everything I had eaten in the past two days, what I had touched or inhaled. When I met with my doctor, I brought my notes. I was certain that the reaction was prompted by the cuts I suffered from the rose thorns. I felt that the thorns had pierced my fingers and micro doses of plant secretion had permeated my system and acted like a poison to me.

My doctor disagreed. The results from my allergy test were available three weeks later. I was told that the "perpetrator" of the allergy was street and domestic dust, but what about the roses and its thorns? No one knows because the test was performed to check only one allergen—dust, probably the most popular one.

My doctor prescribed two bottles of Zyrtec tablets and three bottles of Flonase nasal spray. These two drugs are well-known brands for allergies that are heavily advertised on television.

Since childhood I have been conditioned not to use chemical drugs and to opt for natural remedies instead. I try to avoid chemical medicines as much as possible. I believe in the power of Nature and her green wonders: herbs, fruits, vegetables, homemade elixirs, libations, infusions, poultices, and essential oils. I trust the wisdom of preventive measures and try to keep myself at my best.

However, since I did develop a skin rash, which was rapidly worsening, I had no choice but to resort to taking Zyrtec—60 tablets in 60 days—and Flonase—three nasal sprays for three months. Total expense: $320.00.

That could buy a lot of herbs, fruits, vegetables, and juices, and I could be enjoying those tasty delights instead of chemical wonders. By the way, Zyrtec helped, I must admit. The skin rash disappeared, but gastric upsets appeared, evidently as a side effect. Flonase, on the other hand, did not reduce nasal mucus or the sneezing I experienced. So I have become a "participant" in furthering the prosperity of the pharmaceutical industry. Now I must do a little planning to keep myself out of trouble and bring my body back into balance.

First of all, I begin with a proper diet. I have found that a breakfast consisting of organic farmer's cheese with organic sour cream and honey and lots of hot green tea works for me. You can make mouthwatering, tasty farmer's cheese at home. You'll never find the same in any store. It is so juicy that you don't need to add sour cream. Try it with fresh raspberries for a delicious breakfast, accompanied with hot green tea with jasmine or a mix of Indian and Ceylon tea.

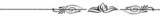

 3. Make fine homemade farmer's cheese. Pour two cartons (you decide how much you want to make) of organic buttermilk into a saucepan and bring to boil. When the whey appears on the surface of the buttermilk, remove from the stove and let it cool off. Then pour it into a large bowl lined with large cheesecloth (washed). Carefully gather the ends of the cheesecloth containing the buttermilk and tie it with a knot. Hang it on your kitchen faucet, allowing the whey to trickle down to the last drop. Your homemade cheese is then ready to eat. Separate into four portions. Eat one part and store the rest in your refrigerator for up to seven days.

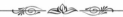

Farmer's cheese gives you a fair dose of calcium to keep bones and teeth strong and balances the metabolism, which creates a solid foundation to help resist allergies.

You can add hot oatmeal to your breakfast menu to clean blood vessels and impart a healthy, fresh appearance to your skin. I have observed for many years that people who suffer from an allergy also suffer from a calcium deficiency, so to keep allergies at bay, it is a good idea to maintain the proper level of calcium in our bodies.

4. Every two to three days make one glass (eight ounces) of fresh carrot juice and drink (chew as if you were chewing food) it before any meal. Parsley can be added to carrot juice as a strong blood purifier.

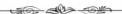

 5. Eat your homemade cheese or three ounces of organic farmer's cheese, all natural, no salt added. It contains vitamins A and C, calcium, and iron. Add one tablespoon of organic sour cream. Mix it and eat as is, or add fresh berries, raisins, and one teaspoon of honey or cherry preserves.

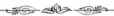

 6. Make one cup of hot green tea with orange, passion fruit and jasmine, Earl Grey, English Breakfast, Prince of Wales, or Ceylon with orange pekoe.

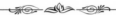

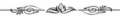

 7. Make one glass of hot chamomile tea and drink it to wash out impurities in the blood vessels.

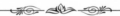

 8. Make a hot oatmeal kasha with a banana sliced into it. Drink a cup of hot herbal tea along with it.

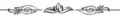

Usually in allergy treatments doctors recommend strong drugs or steroids. I do not recommend such strong measures, but prefer instead alternative medicine.

The following are Russian folk remedies that can help you strengthen and clean the immune and respiratory systems from toxins so allergens will not find a beneficial environment in which to "blossom" into allergic diseases.

Vitamin teas:

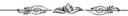

 9. Combine one teaspoon black currants (fresh or dry) and one teaspoon rose hips (fresh or dry) in a glass pitcher with two cups boiling water. Steep for one hour, filter, and add one teaspoon honey. Drink four ounces three to four times a day.

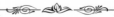

10. Mix one teaspoon black currants, two teaspoons nettle leaf, and three teaspoons rose hips. Follow directions in #9.

 11. Wash two pounds of fresh black currant berries and put into an enamel bowl. Add two pounds of sugar. Mix, rub with a wooden spoon, and mix again. Store in refrigerator, and eat one teaspoon every day or add to hot tea. This mixture keeps vitamins, including vitamin C, fresh for a long time.

Herbal compositions in hot teas

 12. one teaspoon rose hips
one teaspoon black currants

 13. one teaspoon rose hips
one teaspoon cranberries

 14. one teaspoon rose hips
one teaspoon blueberries

15. three teaspoons nettle leaves
three teaspoons blueberries
three teaspoons rose hips

 16. seven teaspoons mountain ash berries
three teaspoons nettle leaves

 17. one teaspoon rose hips
one teaspoon mountain ash berries

Put one tablespoon of herbs and berries in a pot. Add one cup of water and boil for 10 minutes. Steep for four hours and then cover with a small cloth to keep this liquid warm. Take ½ of a glass two to three times a day.

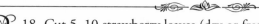

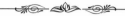

18. Cut 5–10 strawberry leaves (dry or fresh) into small pieces. Add one cup boiling water. Steep for 10–15 minutes and drink as a vitamin tea.

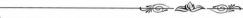

Restoration remedies

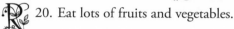

19. Thinly slice two lemons and place layer by layer in a glass jar. Add raw brown sugar or honey to cover each layer of lemon. Eat three to four pieces every day.

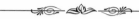

20. Eat lots of fruits and vegetables.

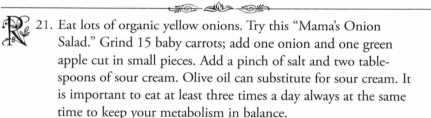

21. Eat lots of organic yellow onions. Try this "Mama's Onion Salad." Grind 15 baby carrots; add one onion and one green apple cut in small pieces. Add a pinch of salt and two table-spoons of sour cream. Olive oil can substitute for sour cream. It is important to eat at least three times a day always at the same time to keep your metabolism in balance.

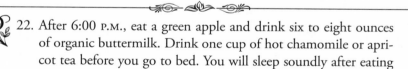

22. After 6:00 P.M., eat a green apple and drink six to eight ounces of organic buttermilk. Drink one cup of hot chamomile or apri-cot tea before you go to bed. You will sleep soundly after eating lightly in the evening.

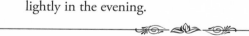

23. Try to fall asleep between 10:00 P.M. and 11:00 P.M. to assure that you get a good sound sleep for at least eight hours. This is enough to restore your nervous system and energy for the next day.

By following the above suggestions, you can say that you have done the best you can in preventing allergic irritants from making you sick. The following is a list of remedies to use when prevention measures fail.

Ailments: allergic skin blisters, spots, red swellings, rashes, eczema, acne.

Remedies:

Cabbage is the first and easiest useful natural tool in emergencies. Cabbage has been used since Dioscorides' time to treat skin and digestive problems, fevers, muscle aches, varicose veins, chronic bowel syndrome, and mastitis. It is known in folk medicine as colewort, which was always ready as a natural medicine for all family sicknesses for many generations.

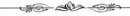

 24. Cut a fresh leaf from a head of cabbage. Wash, beat the leaf to soften, and bind it to the affected area with gauze.

 25. Take ¼ head of cabbage, cut into strips, and put into juicer. Pour fresh cabbage juice into a clean glass bottle or jar. Soak a cotton ball in the juice and apply to the irritated part of skin, a wound, or arthritic joints.

 26. Make cabbage lotion for acne. Mix in a blender ½ pound of fresh cabbage leaves and one tablespoon of olive oil. Strain and add two drops of fresh lemon juice. Soak a cotton ball in your homemade lotion and rub the parts of the face with acne twice a day, once in the morning and once in the evening.

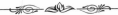

27. Onion can be successfully substituted for cabbage. Cut an onion and place a thin rounded piece on the affected area. It will relieve allergic rash (nettle rash) caused by food allergens.

We know that celery is a nourishing vegetable, but it is also a useful medicinal plant because it has antitoxic properties and it is a restorative and cleansing tonic for allergic conditions and in arthritis, kidney diseases, and nervous exhaustion. It can serve as a natural cleanser, diuretic, laxative, and energy booster.

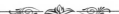

 28. Make fresh juice from celery leaves, root, and stalks. Take two teaspoons three times a day 30 minutes before you go to bed.

 29. Make celery infusion. Crush two tablespoons of celery roots. Add eight ounces of cold spring water and steep for two hours. Filter and drink three ounces two to three times daily before a meal.

 30. Make fresh cranberry juice. Drink four to eight ounces a day. Soak gauze in the juice and apply to the area affected by allergic rash, eczema, sores, or pimples.

 31. Add 12 ounces of boiling water to one ounce of freshly dried hops. Steep for 30 minutes, filter, and drink four ounces a day before meals.

 32. Combine in an enamel pot one tablespoon St. John's Wort, one tablespoon eyebright, one tablespoon dandelion root, one tablespoon horsetail, ½ teaspoon corn silk, one tablespoon chamomile, and 1½ tablespoons rose hips. Add five cups boiling water, steep eight hours, and then warm to boiling. Filter and drink three ounces three times a day before meals. Continue for six months. This natural medicine remains fresh in the refrigerator for up to three days. Make a fresh batch again after that.

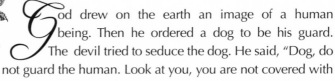

God drew on the earth an image of a human being. Then he ordered a dog to be his guard. The devil tried to seduce the dog. He said, "Dog, do not guard the human. Look at you, you are not covered with anything, but I will give you a good fur coat, and you'll feel fine and warm."

The dog was confused, but he went away from the human's image, which was drawn by God. When the devil saw that the dog had left the human, he grabbed a spear, struck the drawing of the man with it, and inflicted him with 70 wounds.

When God saw what the devil had done, he created 70 medicinal herbs to heal these wounds.

Remedies:

The treatment of eczema, as one of the complicated forms of allergy and skin disorders, can be very effective with a proper preparation and the use of herbal medicines. Be patient; sometimes excellent results will appear after several months of treatment.

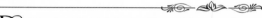

 33. Avoid drinking coffee or black tea for several years if you want to get rid of allergic reactions. Instead drink spring water and herbal teas.

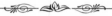

 34. Take an agrimony *(Agrimonia eupatoria)* bath. Combine four ounces of agrimony with one quart of boiling water and steep for 20 minutes. Add to your bathtub and enjoy. In the fifteenth century this healing herb was the prime remedy for gunshot wounds on the battlefield. Agrimony has been used since Saxon times to treat wounds.

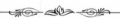

 35. The combination of oak bark, calendula (pot marigold), and yarrow is also a good healing remedy for eczema sores.

    a) Place one teaspoon of agrimony in a mug. Add boiling water and steep for five minutes.

    b) Place one teaspoon of yarrow in a mug. Add boiling water and steep for seven minutes.

    c.) Place one tablespoon of crushed oak bark in an enamel pot. Add one quart of water and bring to a boil. Add four ounces of agrimony tea and four ounces of yarrow tea in a pot with boiling oak bark liquid. Mix with a wooden spoon. Boil for two minutes. Remove from the stove and steep for 15 minutes. When the liquid has cooled but is still warm, soak your hand with eczema sore inside the pot and keep there until the herbal medicine becomes cold. Don't dry your hand with a towel. Allow to air dry.

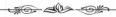

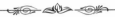

 36. Place one tablespoon of nettle leaves and stems in an enamel pot with one cup of boiling water. Cover with a lid and wrap with a warm fabric. Steep for 30 minutes, filter, and drink four ounces four to five times a day or eight ounces of warm nettle infusion three times a day.

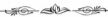

This natural medicine is an excellent blood purifier and it helps to heal allergic rash, itch, eczema, and other skin disorders. Nettle is a well-known folk remedy. It stimulates blood circulation and cleanses the body when people suffer eczema, rheumatism, or arthritis. It can also increase milk flow in nursing mothers. This herb absorbs many minerals from the soil and contains a high percent of vitamin C, which helps the body to adjust these minerals, especially iron.

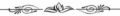

 37. Place one tablespoon each of nettle, agrimony, strawberry leaves, and heartsease into an enamel pot with one quart of boiling water. Steep overnight in a preheated but cooling oven. In the morning filter and warm the mixture. Drink one cup three times a day. This herbal mixture is an effective healer of allergic rash and pimples. It is an excellent cleanser, especially in food intolerance which provokes different diseases where a blood purifier is needed such as digestive upsets, kidney illnesses, childhood anemia, congestion, skin rashes, urinary infections, and respiratory problems.

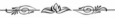

 38. Duckweed nastoyka (infusion) is used to treat almost all allergic conditions, especially skin rashes and swelling of a nervous origin. Wash fresh duckweed plant. Put one teaspoon in a glass jar. Add 50 ml (two ounces) vodka. Seal the jar and store in a cool place for seven days. Stir occasionally. Filter into a pitcher. With your fingers press the mixture through cheesecloth to extract more liquid. Then pour the strained liquid into a pre-washed dark glass bottle. Use a funnel if necessary. Pour 15-20 drops of tincture into two ounces of water and take three times a day. Any part of the plant can be used in nastoykas with vodka. This method offers two benefits:

a.) All active ingredients are extracted.

b) Vodka is a natural preservative, so nastoyka/tincture can be used for two years, if stored in a cool place.

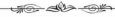

> **Ailments:** allergic rhinitis, nasal mucus, sneezing, hay fever, conjunctivitis, allergic asthma, provoked by plants; trees; flowers pollens; hay, street, house, and bookshelf dust; or animal hair.

Remedies:

 39. Make or buy fresh birch juice and drink it for one month as a substitute for water or tea.

 40. Mary's Root powder. Wash a dry peony root. Dry, and grind it to a powder. Take three tablespoons a day 30 minutes before a meal. This effectively treats allergic rhinitis because the root's bark is a good antibacterial and it can be used to heal more complicated illnesses such as abscesses, skin inflammations, eczema, liver disorders, and nervous conditions. This powder (1½ tablespoons a day) can be used to treat children with a strong allergic rhinitis. This condition can be fully treated in three to five days if peony powder is taken regularly as prescribed. If a child doesn't like the taste of this powder, mix it with cherry or apricot preserves and offer it with a cup of hot water, sweetened with honey.

 41. Place one tablespoon of Greater celandine aerial parts in a large glass jar. Add two glasses of boiling water. Let steep for three hours. Take two to four ounces twice a day, once in the morning and once in the evening. This herb is an anti-inflammatory, diuretic and cleanser, and a liver stimulant. **Avoid in pregnancy.**

 42. Grind to a powder burdock and dandelion roots. Mix well and place two tablespoons of the mixture into a glass jar. Add 24 ounces of cold boiled water and steep overnight. In the morning boil the liquid for 10 minutes and steep for an additional 10 minutes. Drink four ounces four to five times a day before any meal and before you go to bed.

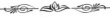

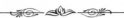

 43. Grind dried duckweed to a powder. Mix it with honey in equal proportions. Take two grams of the mixture twice a day.

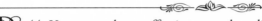

 44. You can make an effective natural medicine from the blossoms of the Self-Heal (Prunella vulgaris) plant. Dry the plant in the sun and grind the blossoms to a powder. Take one tablespoon three times a day with hot tea.

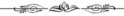

 45. Make Self-Heal nastoyka. Combine one tablespoon of Self-Heal powder with eight ounces of boiling water. Steep for three to five minutes and drink hot.

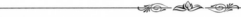

 46. Combine one tablespoon chamomile flowers in a glass jar with eight ounces boiling water. Step for 10 minutes. Take one tablespoon four times a day.

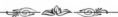

 47. Combine one tablespoon of calendula (pot marigold) with four ounces boiling water. Steep for one hour. Take one tablespoon three times a day.

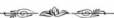

 48. Combine one tablespoon of peppermint leaves with four ounces of boiling water. Steep for 20 minutes. Take one tablespoon three times a day.

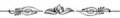

 49. Combine two tablespoons of nettle with two cups boiling water. Steep for two hours. Drink two ounces four times a day before meals.

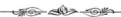

Remedies:

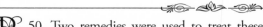

50. Two remedies were used to treat these conditions in our family. Grandma made her nastoyka Black Knight to treat skin problems.

    Put one teaspoon crushed black currant leaves in a teapot and pour two cups boiling water over the leaves. Let it infuse for four hours and then strain through a nylon sieve into a pitcher. Store in a cool place. Add a wedge of fresh lemon and take ½ cup four times a day.

    Eat plenty of fresh gooseberries. The medicinal properties of these berries are very effective in the treatment of skin problems, because they contain vitamins A, B, C and bioflavonoids which help to improve circulation and strengthen the capillaries to free the skin of allergic reactions.

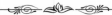

51. Rinse throat with herbal infusions, using valerian root to calm the nervous system. Combine one teaspoon of valerian root with two cups boiling water. Steep for 10 minutes. Rinse the throat once a day in the evening. Keep the remaining infusion in the refrigerator up to three days but no longer.

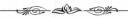

52. Make infusion with motherwort herb. Use the same method of preparation as in #51.

53. Take a shower three times a day to open pores and cleanse all systems from toxins accumulated in the body.

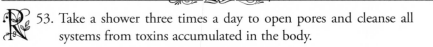

54. Make a compress for the eyes by infusing two tea bags of black tea in eight ounces of boiling water. Steep for 10 minutes and allow cooling. Soak two cotton balls in the warm tea and place them on irritated eyes for three minutes. Continue treatment for three to five days.

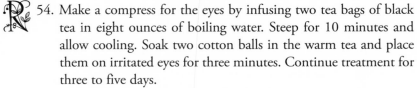

Sunlight and hot and cold temperatures can sometimes be irritants that assist the body in forming harmful substances that become allergens, but sunlight can also change the colors around us: yellow into orange, light green into forest green, light blue into navy, purple into lavender, pink into red, and red into fire-orange. In folk medicine colors are often used to promote healing.

> **Ailments:** irritated, blurry eyes; loss of energy; "hot" head; headache; skin rash.

Remedies:

When sunbeams pass through a glass of different colors, they can be an effective treatment for various ailments, including those of the skin and eyes. This is described in the oldest world science—astrology. Keep an open mind and let's explore this further. In an ancient Indian manuscript, astrology is described as "a natural daughter, born of a liaison and love of strong numbers and perspicacious intuition." Intuition told astrologers, and experimentation confirmed to scientists, that when sunbeams pass through a glass, they become a healing energy. This was considered in astrology as a display of one of the laws of Mother Nature.

Sunbeams contain a spectrum of seven colors, given in accordance with the seven planets:

Red — Mars

Navy — Venus

Yellow — Mercury

Green — Saturn

Purple — Jupiter

Orange — Sun

Violet — Moon

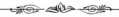

 55. **Red**, the color of Mars, is useful in the treatment of inflammatory processes. A person who is suffering from inflammation would be advised to retire to a room where red is the predominant color,

from walls to bedspreads. The sunbeams penetrating that room will also be red. Although many people equate the color red with attention and emergency, according to astrology, it is a natural healer and plays an important role in warning us of diseases such as colds, flu, bronchitis, and pneumonia.

 56. **Navy blue** acts as a sedative for intellectual people who are involved in intensive brainwork. Adding navy blue curtains or a lampshade to a bedroom can be an excellent source of calming and relaxation for people who have weak eyesight or suffer a nervous disorder or mental disease.

 57. **Green** also acts as a sedative and is an especially effective healer for people with irritated, blurry eyes, affected by an allergic reaction.

 58. **Orange** calms the appetite.

 59. **Yellow** acts as a healer for people with intestinal disorders.

 60. **Purple** is useful for treating blood and liver diseases.

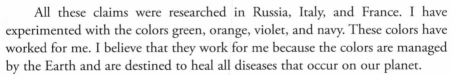 61. **Violet** treats nervous disorders and vegetative neurosis.

All these claims were researched in Russia, Italy, and France. I have experimented with the colors green, orange, violet, and navy. These colors have worked for me. I believe that they work for me because the colors are managed by the Earth and are destined to heal all diseases that occur on our planet.

There is also a principle of sympathy and antipathy concerning these colors and, when we fully understand how this mysterious kaleidoscope of colors work, our optimum health will be the benefit we derive from them. Look how the green color from Mother Nature can work for us.

The Green Savior

Once upon a time a big city gathered so much dust, smoke, and odorous, toxic fumes that the people who lived there could no longer breathe easily. They got sinus infections and nasal drops that their doctors prescribed for them, didn't help at all. Purple and blue violets, pale pink hyacinths, bright yellow daisies, red tulips and carnations, "orange gypsies"—marigolds, white tiger lilies, and creamy climbing roses were asphyxiated by gasoline and died in the city parks and gardens by the thousands.

The blooming bird-cherry trees had dried before the eyes after breathing in the city air. The beautiful tall maples "burned" down. The acorns, poisoned by the city's fumes and smoke, fell down from the powerful gigantic oaks. The red ash-berries on the blossoming rowan trees got sick with allergies from the city dust and pollution.

The citizens complained, "What a mess! How can we rid our city of this pollution? We are sick and no longer have clean air."

They screamed, "Help! Help! Can anyone hear us in this world?"

Their cries awakened a thick, emerald forest that had stood near the city for many years. In an effort to help the desperate people, the forest assembled an army of tree soldiers. Pines, firs, birches, mountain ashes, oaks, and poplars marched into the city in well-proportioned columns, spreading their saving oxygen everywhere. The toxins in the air became panic stricken.

"We cannot breathe anymore! We are dying! The tree soldiers are choking us!" they yelled.

When the dust, toxins, and bacteria smelled the fragrant needles of the pines, they felt strangled and were caught up in a tornado funnel and swept away by the big, leafy, green boughs. The fresh green mist that filled the city carried the scent of a forest in the spring. The heavy, dank, and poisonous air became light and fragrant with the scent of pine, fir, and birch. It was also scented with heavenly jasmine and wild rosemary, thyme, and basil.

The green mist floated into people's houses through the open windows, doors, and keyholes. While the people slept, they began to breathe easier and those who had suffered from sinus infections, flu, sleeplessness and allergies had a sound sleep filled with sweet dreams as never before.

The brave soldiers of the green forest marched through the city, winning one area after another until the city was clean and pure. And even today people are greeted by thousands of fresh junipers; pines; and millions of red, white, and pink geraniums placed at every corner of the city by the green soldiers to guard the people from pollution and sicknesses.

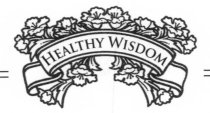

Nature ever flows; stands never still.
Motion or change is her mode of existence.

—*Ralph Waldo Emerson (1802–1882), American poet and essayist*

Junipers on the mountains were thickly hung with berries,
and the air was unadulterated gin.

—*John McPhee (1931–), American writer*

Winds are advertisements of all they touch, however much or little we
may be able to read; telling their wanderings even by their scents alone.

—*John Muir (1838–1914), Scottish-born American naturalist*

Let us a little permit Nature to take her own way;
she better understands her own affairs than we.

—Michel Euquem de Montaigne (1533–1592), French writer

The field has eyes, the wood has ears; I will look, be silent, and listen.

—Hieronymus Bosch (1450–1516), Dutch painter

Shall I not have intelligence with the earth?
Am I not partly leaves and vegetable mould myself?

—Henry David Thoreau (1817–1862), American writer

Besides the motives that have been mentioned, it may be added that the
Great Khan is more disposed to plant trees because astrologers tell him
that those who plant trees are rewarded with long life.

—Marco Polo (1254–1324), Italian merchant and traveler

All my life throught, the new sights of Nature
made me rejoice like a child.

—Marie Curie (1867–1934), Polish-born French chemist

I think that I cannot preserve my health and spirits,
unless I spend four hours a day at least — and it is commonly more
than that — sauntering through the woods and over the hills and fields,
absolutely free from all worldly engagements.

—Henry David Thoreau (1817–1862), American writer

Chapter 6

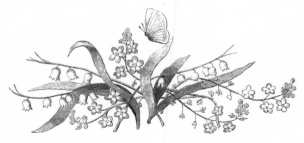

Ourselves, Our Children, Allergens, and Happy Cells

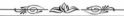

Use the folk medicine recipes in this chapter only
under the guidance of your child's pediatrician.

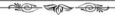

Never put off till tomorrow what you can do today.

—Russian proverb

FACTS

Up to two million or 8 percent of children in the United States are
estimated to be affected by food allergy. If one parent has allergic disease, the
estimated risk of a child to develop allergies is 48 percent. The child's estimated
risk grows to 70 percent if both parents have a history of allergy.[21]

As you know now, allergens are irritating substances that provoke
high sensitivity in the human body. When children are small
(from one month to three years old), allergens that affect them can
be milk, eggs, peanuts, oranges, and strawberries. Later on (ages three and up),
allergens might include medical drugs, detergents, fragrances, weeds, molds

and mildew, substances found in home air ducts, flower pollen, and other substances that penetrate their body through their delicate skin.

Animal dander from the hair of domestic pets including dogs, cats, and rabbits can be allergens on contact, as can bird feathers and fur jackets. Any allergic reaction can develop into illness.

Infants and young children usually become ill more readily than older children and their illness may be more intense. This is because the immune system of an infant or young child is not as developed as that of an older child. Allergies and other ailments contracted by infants and children up to six years old develop fast and have a tendency to spread through the body in a matter of hours. For example, small inflammations (blisters) on an infant's skin may indicate a "general" sickness—sepsis.

Diathesis is a heightened (abnormal) sensitivity of mucous membranes and skin to external irritants. Symptoms usually appear during the first months of a child's life. In the second half of the first year of an infant's life, these signs became much clearer. Some food products show up as diathesis. Closely monitor your child for any reactions from these foods: milk, eggs, cheese, chocolate, cocoa, nuts, oranges, strawberries, soda, or any canned beverages.

Consider that diathesis, provoked by sugar or foods that are rich in carbohydrates, is common as a first allergy. One of the first signs of diathesis, which may appear in the first two or three months of a child's life, is "milk scab," yellowish, crusty patches that form on the child's scalp and above the eyebrows.

Some mothers try to remove these scaly patches only to find that they form again and spread to the baby's cheeks. At first the skin on the cheeks will redden and then become rough to the touch. Dry or wet eczema and its accompanying itching may follow.

Wet eczema is not pretty. First, a rash, which turns to blisters, appears on the skin. These blisters eventually burst, leaving small, wet wounds that dry and form scabs. Dry and wet eczema require different treatments and, once healed, they can return.

Children's skin rashes typically occur from three months to six years of age, especially during spring and summer. Be sure to include an assortment of fruits in your child's diet to afford him the natural vitamins that strengthen the immune system. Remember that organic produce is best because it is not sprayed with pesticides and other chemicals, which can also prompt allergic reactions.

Skin rashes in the form of itchy red bumps or knots may also develop as a result of eating food allergens. Usually these red knots find a comfortable place in the nooks and crannies of the upper and lower extremities.

Some children may exhibit a high sensitivity of the mucous membranes of the nose and throat, irritation of the genitals and/or conjunctivitis, an inflammation of the mucous membranes of the eyes. The structure and color of the tongue and its mucous membranes change dramatically from red to white.

The occurrences of exudative diathesis may remind one of ocean waves, rolling by turns to the shore. Many children maintain clear, clean skin between the periods of acute conditions, and when children reach the age of two or three, the skin rashes disappear as suddenly as they appeared. But children are vulnerable and may experience respiratory reactions to allergens. They might develop bronchitis or bronchial asthma, due to the lack of appropriate medical treatment at the proper time.

A friend of mine has two sons who were born five years apart. Both suffered a harsh form of exudative diathesis from one month old up to four years old. Skin rashes developed behind their ears in the form of wet, blistered eczema. When the blisters burst, they left small, bleeding wounds. It took several weeks for these wounds to dry and heal.

Then two to three weeks later the condition reappeared. The two boys suffered this diathesis for four years with antiseptic baths and time being the only remedies.

Children with diathesis need special care and attention

 1. Use only natural fabrics such as cotton blankets and diapers for your baby.

 2. Cloth should be soft and able to "breathe."

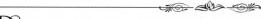 3. Use a mild, unscented natural soap to wash anything that comes in contact with your child.

 4. Detect food products that provoke allergic reactions in your child and exclude them.

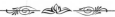

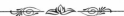

5. If your child is food sensitive, introduce foods one at a time, every week in turns, to detect more easily which one prompts an allergic reaction.

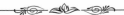

6. I believe that it is helpful to substitute organic buttermilk or organic kefir as an alternative to milk. When your child is three months old, give him homemade vegetable puree. Consult a physician specializing in the treatment of allergies if a reaction occurs.

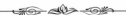

7. Every child requires individualized treatment based on his or her allergies and environment.

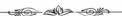

8. Give your child a massage. It will make him/her stronger to fight diseases.

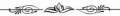

9. Give your child a seated bath twice a day with chamomile or calendula (pot marigold). Put one tablespoon of chamomile flowers or calendula into a cup. Add boiling water. Infuse for 10 minutes. Then pass it through strainer or nylon sieve and pour this liquid into the bath water.

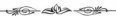

10. Make a pink bath. Add one tiny pinch of potassium permanganate to the warm bath water to create a pale rose color. It is an excellent antiseptic and keeps a child's skin clean and healthy.

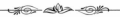

11. Combine one teaspoon each of chamomile, calendula, and oak bark with one quart of boiling water. Let steep for 10 minutes, filter, and pour into a warm bath. Bathe your child for 15 minutes.

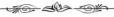

12. Combine a pinch of potassium permanganate and boric acid with two cups of warm water. Soak a swatch of soft cotton in this light pink liquid and apply as a compress to wet eczema.

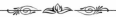

Allergy and colds

Children prone to allergic reactions often get sick with colds. Prepare them to fight it.

---

 13. Combine one quart of water with one teaspoon of sea salt, five drops of iodine, and two to three tablespoons of vodka. Soak a swatch of soft cotton in this lotion to rub on your child once in the morning during the cold seasons of the year. Later bathe the child in a warm bath. The lotion will nourish your child's skin and help him/her to fight allergy and colds.

Here are folk remedies that heal skin rashes and improve metabolism.

---

 14. Mince one teaspoon dandelion root and combine with one cup boiling water in a glass jar. Seal and cover with a warm fabric. Steep for one to five hours, filter into a pitcher, and store in a cool place. Take two tablespoons three to four times a day 30 minutes before meals.

---

 15. Mince one tablespoon burdock root and combine with ½ quart boiling water in a large glass jar. Seal and cover with flannel or wool fabric to keep it warm. Steep for one to five hours, filter into a pitcher, and store in a cool place. Warm and drink ½ cup three to four times a day. This is a strong blood purifier and effective cleanser for children and adults, especially when excess toxins create skin problems, arthritic pains, and digestive sluggishness.

---

 16. Use the infusion in #15 to treat skin rashes, sores, and infections externally by applying a burdock compress to the affected area.

---

 17. Give your child several glasses of spring water to drink every day. Add a slice of organic lemon, apple or quince to make it more appealing. This helps to fight allergic reactions associated with

colds or food allergies. Quince juice can help rid the system of toxins and is also effective when applied externally to skin disorders.

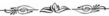

18. Add two cups of boiling water to one tablespoon of dried agrimony leaves. Infuse for 8–10 minutes. Strain and pour into a glass jar. Use this infusion to wash sores, wounds, eczema or soak a sterile pad in the infusion and apply to the affected area. This herb provides an effective treatment for children suffering from diathesis and eczema.

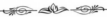

19. To four cups boiling water, add one tablespoon licorice root, 1½ tablespoons dandelion root, and 1½ tablespoons burdock root. Steep for 30 minutes and strain. Children may take two to four ounces twice a day. Adults may take 8–16 ounces twice a day, in the morning and in the evening.

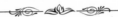

20. To ½ quart of boiling water, add one teaspoon each of elecampane root, gentian herb, and yarrow and steep for 30 minutes. Take one tablespoon three times a day for one to two months before meals.

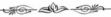

21. Prepare this natural medicine, using the same method as in #18. Add the water to ½ tablespoon diced licorice root and ½ tablespoon diced heartsease. Drink up to one cup a day. Always remember to complement all treatments with fresh organic fruit or vegetable salads after dinner.

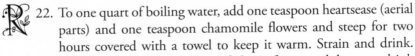

22. To one quart of boiling water, add one teaspoon heartsease (aerial parts) and one teaspoon chamomile flowers and steep for two hours covered with a towel to keep it warm. Strain and drink. Children may take **only** ⅓ of this infusion; adults may drink three times a day.

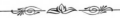

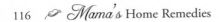

All allergic conditions

Internal use:

 23. Make strawberry liquor (for age one and up). Combine eight ounces of dried or fresh strawberries with one pint of water and one tablespoon of honey or unrefined sugar in a saucepan. Stir constantly over medium heat until dissolved. Boil it to reduce by half, cool, and pour into a dark glass bottle. Seal with a cork stopper. Do not use a screw-capped lid because liquors and syrups ferment in closed bottles and can explode. Children may take one teaspoon two or three times a day.

 24. Make a chamomile infusion. Add eight ounces boiling water to one tablespoon chamomile flowers. Steep in a glass pitcher for 20 minutes. Take one tablespoon three to four times daily.

 25. Try a peppermint infusion. Add one tablespoon peppermint leaves to ½ cup boiling water. Cover and steep for 20 minutes. Take one tablespoon three times a day.

 26. To make a simple calendula (pot marigold) infusion, add one tablespoon calendula flowers to four ounces boiling water. Steep for one hour. Take one tablespoon two to three times daily.

 27. Eggshell powder. Carefully and thoroughly wash three to four eggs (organic/free-range chicken eggs). Boil them for 10 minutes. Cool and peel eggshell from membrane, then grind into powder in glass, stone, or ceramic bowl. Use a mortar and pestle. Never use a metal bowl. Before you give one pinch of eggshell powder to your child, add five drops of natural lemon juice.

- A baby six months to one year old takes ¼ teaspoon of eggshell powder.
- A child 1–1½ years old takes ⅓ teaspoon.
- Children from 1½–2 years take ½ teaspoon.

The eggshell powder healing process is a long one, but there is another benefit; it contains a significant amount of calcium. In any case, it can be taken from several weeks to a month until the allergy is eliminated, but even over time the method is harmless.

---

28. Young nettle usually bears juicy leaves in April or May, depending on its geographical location. Cut the upper 10 inches of nettle stem with leaves. Wash well and dice, then place the pieces in a one-quart glass jar filled to the top with cold boiled water. Leave it to infuse for eight hours. Give a child this infusion blended with various juices or compotes of fresh cherries, cranberries, or gooseberries. This effective and tasty treatment cleans allergens from the blood and calms the digestive and nervous systems.

I believe in miracles! Herbal baths effectively treat almost all allergic reactions that you or your children might have. As I mentioned earlier, a bath with a tiny addition of potassium permanganate has effectively treated many generations of children.

Herbal infusions positively affect the skin and the whole body through it. If you use the appropriate herbs in the correct dosage, a bath with an herbal addition is a true blessing. It will restore the normal function of the skin and destroy pathogenic microbes. It helps rid the body of toxins. Herbal baths can soothe a child's and an adult's nervous system.

Rejuvenating baths for children and adults include such dried herbs and plants as chamomile (flowers), thyme or wild marjoram (aerial parts), nettle (aerial parts, roots), oats (grain), horsetail (aerial parts), strawberry (leaves), and rose hips (berries).

A special tonic/herbal series of bath therapies: six to eight baths for 10–20 minutes each will restore, nourish, and support the entire body and protect it from germs and allergens. Bath time should be no longer than 15–20 minutes. When you take an herbal bath, do not use any soap. It will destroy the medicinal properties of the herbs.

Key:

Children up to 15 years old: ½ pound of herbs to one gallon of cold water and ½ pound of herbs for a decoction. Adults: two gallons of cold water and 1½ pounds of herbs.

For each of the following herbal bath recipes, use two to five ounces of each herb. Boil the mixture for 10–15 minutes. Steep for 30 minutes, strain, pour into the bathtub, and add water as needed.

 29. Chamomile, nettle, oats (blossoming), heartsease, and thyme.

 30. Rose petals and leaves of black currant and strawberry.

 31. Nettle, birch leaves, heartsease, and wild marjoram.

 32. Horsetail, nettle, oats and rose hips, in equal proportions up to 100 grams or about four ounces.

Rejuvenating baths for children

 33. Dice two ounces juniper twigs and add to one quart cold water. Steep for one hour and then boil for 15 minutes. Strain and relax in a warm bath before a night's sleep. Take a series of 12 baths for the best results.

 34. In a cotton bag, mix four tablespoons oak bark, one tablespoon wild marjoram, one tablespoon yarrow flowers, one tablespoon pine twigs with needles, one tablespoon heartsease flowers and stems, one pound black currant leaves, one pound wheat bran, and one pound rye flowers. Place the bag in a large pot of water (up to 10 gallons). Simmer for 45 minutes. Use all this decoction for one bath.

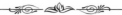

 35. Mix one tablespoon each chamomile flowers and thyme; 1½ tablespoons each wild marjoram, oak leaves, black currant leaves, and sage leaves; two tablespoons each burdock root and pine buds; one pound wheat siftings or bran; and ½ pound rye flowers. Boil 25 minutes in two gallons of water. Strain and pour into a bathtub. Add warm water as needed. Bathe for 15 minutes. This infusion helps to treat diathesis, and children with weakened immune systems who are readily exposed to infectious ailments in schools and other public places.

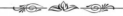

 36. Mix one tablespoon birch leaves, two tablespoons wild marjoram, and three tablespoons nettle leaves. The method of preparation is the same as in #35.

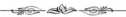

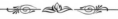 37. Mix five tablespoons chamomile, three tablespoons black currant leaves, and two tablespoons thyme. The method of preparation is the same as in #35. This composition of herbs is a strong disinfectant. It helps to calm and restore the nervous system and stimulates the metabolism.

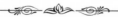

 38. Combine two tablespoons wild marjoram, five tablespoons nettle leaves, four tablespoons each chamomile and horsetail. The method of preparation is the same as in #35.

Such herbs as lemon balm, borage, echinacea, evening primrose, ginseng, nettles, and aromatherapy oils melissa and chamomile can be used too as a treatment of allergies.

We do not have to go far from the houses we live in to suffer from allergies. Some common household allergens include dust, pet dander, aquarium fish food, cleaning products—the list is seemingly endless.

So what can we do? Move to the moon? Travel to Venus? Shut ourselves into a sterile box? The first thing we do is relax. The answer lies in natural remedies. It could be acupuncture; fresh air; medicinal herbs, plants, and trees; or spending time in Nature that cures our ills.

Our attitudes can also play a big part in how we perceive our suffering. Try the following suggestions to alleviate a grim outlook:

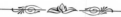

 39. Sing merry, melodic songs to yourself and to your children.

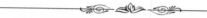

 40. Sing songs together with your children. Singing is a pleasant natural treatment for allergy too. Our skin cells are good listeners because our skin is a "buffer" between the human body and the surrounding world. They absorb good and bad influences like parched earth absorbs water. Our millions of body cells protect us from irritants (invaders), but if we fail to take care of them, they cannot defend us from illnesses.

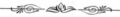

When we practice a proper diet and lifestyle and take time out to soak in an herbal bath, our skin cells react positively to our good actions. We may not notice that sometimes we begin to sing as our head rests on a bath pillow.

Our skin cells thank us for keeping them clean, healthy, and free from illnesses. Our skin cells even smile at us. You find that hard to believe? Come to the mirror and take a good look at your children or at yourself after a cleansing, relaxing, or invigorating herbal bath. You can see how the herbs and water and quiet time have removed the lines of stress from your face and how your skin glows with a renewed radiance. You are happy with the way you look! Your children look rested and refreshed, squeaky clean, and content.

Do you remember the fairy tale of the wicked queen with the magic mirror?

"You are the fairest one of all," the mirror told the wicked queen.

Then one day she became old and ugly because she did not want to do anything good—she did not even want to take a healthy and wholesome herbal bath.

Do not wait until "one day." Fill your bathtub with pre-washed fresh petals of red damask rose and breathe in a delicate smell of this most sensuous of flowers, praised by poets and artists for centuries as a symbol of beauty and love. According to Greek myth, Three Graces gave the rose charm, brightness, and joy; the goddess of love, Aphrodite, gave beauty; the god of wine, Dionysus, added sweet nectar to create an enchanting scent. The wind god, Zephyr, blew the clouds especially for her, the Queen of Flowers, so she could open her petals to the sun and blossom under a flow of the radiant rays of the rising sun.

Long ago ancient Romans also told the world how the red rose got its color. When Jupiter caught Venus bathing naked, she was confused and blushed, and the white rose turned red in her reflection. The Persians created another legend telling that the rose was a great inspiration for a nightingale. The bird began to sing when roses first blossomed, and overcome by their strong aroma a nightingale dropped to the earth. Its spilled blood stained the white rose petals and turned them red.

Since ancient times, the rose was praised not only for its beauty and aroma but also for its medicinal properties. Pliny listed more than 32 remedies made from roses. Avicenna highly valued rose in his practice and was the first to make rose water. Russian Empress Catherine the Great loved roses very much and made her own rose water, which she added in combination with rose petals to her baths for her joy and to cleanse and tone her skin and prevent wrinkles. Probably she knew well that both the leaves and petals of roses clear from the body toxins and heat which produce rashes, itch, and inflammatory problems.

So again, don't wait until "one day."

Mix your special herbal bath now, add pre-washed fresh petals of the red rose, and slide down into the bath water. Rest your head on a pillow and let the herbs do their wondrous work of removing harmful toxins from your skin cells and soothing your spirit. While you are relaxing and listening to beautiful music, you can read this Russian folk tale about one amazing scarlet flower which brought love and happiness to one young girl. I told it to my children in my own interpretation and they liked it very much.

*O*nce upon a time in a far-away land lived one very successful merchant. He traveled many times a year to all parts of the world to sell his goods. He also brought home nice gifts to his three daughters from his travels.

This time he was going to leave for a long journey into a country no one had ever heard of. Before his departure, the merchant came to his three daughters to say goodbye and asked them what gifts they would like him to bring from his voyage. The first daughter, Pasha, asked him to bring her a gold crown. The second daughter, Dasha, wanted a crystal mirror, and the third and youngest daughter, Masha, asked modestly for a little scarlet flower.

The merchant left for his voyage. As soon as his journey began, he easily found a beautiful golden crown for his older daughter and a fine crystal mirror for his second daughter. However, he couldn't find anywhere the gift for his youngest daughter, the scarlet flower. He was looking everywhere and couldn't find it until he entered a beautiful emerald green forest. He kept walking, and the forest's narrow path brought him to a magnificent white palace built right in the center of the forest. He walked inside through the tall wrought-iron black with gold gate and found himself in the spacious courtyard with a blooming flowerbed in the middle of it. On the top of the flowerbed he saw a beautiful flower growing there. He had never seen a similar one anywhere.

The merchant approached closer to the flower and saw it was the scarlet flower his third daughter, Masha, wanted so badly. He picked up the flower carefully, and suddenly he was confronted by a hideous beast. The beast was very angry and said to the merchant, "If you want this flower, you must send one of your daughters back to my enchanted forest to live in my palace forever."

Afraid, the merchant agreed. Soon he returned home and gave the gifts to his two daughters. Then he gave the scarlet flower to his youngest daughter and told her that she had to return a favor for having this rare flower and go to the beast. Masha was so happy that her father had found the scarlet flower that she agreed to go alone to the emerald forest and live forever in the beast's palace.

The next day Masha went to the forest to live in the beast's palace. Several servants met her there and helped her settle in, but the beast himself didn't show up. However, every day he sent her beautiful fresh roses and gifts. One day he sent her a funny-speaking red-blue parrot; another day, a merry brownish-orange monkey. The third day he gave her a tiny, cute white puppy. Then she got from the beast a beautiful grey pony with yellow spots, so she could ride around the palace in the green grassy meadows shining with small drops of the morning dew.

The beast and his servants took very good care of Masha, and she felt loved. She was happy to live in the palace, but she always wondered what the mysterious beast looked like. She never saw him. In the morning she walked in the garden blossoming with white and pink peonies, yellow and red roses, puffy carnations, purple violets and daisies, and tall sunflowers. She enjoyed the beauties of Nature and the sunny, warm days. In the afternoons she swam in the crystal glass pool with sky-blue water. In the evenings before she went to sleep, she took rejuvenating baths filled with lavender and aromatic petals of freshly cut red roses.

Life was good, but all this was not enough for the curious Masha. Every day she wondered about the mysterious beast. What did he look like? One day she asked the servants to let the beast know that she would like to see him. She was very sad this day because the night before she had a bad dream that her father was seriously sick.

In the morning after a walk in the garden she was sitting near the big window in the palace hall thinking about her ill father, her mother, and her sisters she missed so much. Suddenly she heard a light noise that sounded like oak tree leaves were murmuring with each other or wanted to tell her something. After that the beast appeared in front of her in a blink of an eye. The girl was terrified. The beast was a big, ugly man with sharp, cold eyes looking at her and waiting for her to say something. At first Masha couldn't say a word because of her fear.

Then she said, "Dear beast, I am very grateful for all your gifts and the opportunity to live in your magnificent castle. Last night I had a very bad dream that my beloved father got very sick and can die any minute. Please let me go to see him while he's still alive. Maybe I can heal him."

The beast looked at her unhappily and said, "Okay, you can go, my gorgeous girl, but remember you must come back precisely on the third day not later than midnight or something bad may happen."

"I'll be back exactly as you ask," Masha promised.

When she arrived home, she found her mother and her sisters in good health, but her father was very sick as she has seen him in her dream. She prepared for him her magic remedies from the herbs she picked up in the beast's garden. She cooked for her father delicious meals and fed him herself spoon by spoon like he was her small child. She even slept every night near his bed in a small armchair and watched him every minute. Under Masha's loving care her sick father recovered fast.

Three days passed as one minute, and Masha was still there in her parents' house. She didn't notice the time and she didn't know that her sisters, happy that she was taking good care of their father, changed the time on the clock. So Masha stayed one day more before she found out about her sisters' trick with the clock. She was late to return to the beast's palace. In the meantime she was very happy that she had healed her father, but she was very unhappy that she didn't keep her promise to the beast. She was scared that something bad might happen, as the beast told her. She said goodbye to her father in a hurry and ran back to the emerald forest with the speed of the fastest young doe.

She was out of breath when she entered the beast's palace. She feared the punishment she would encounter from the beast. To her great surprise, she found the beast dead, lying on the shiny marble floor in the grand ballroom. He was holding in his hand her favorite scarlet flower. Masha's eyes filled with tears. She was horrified and heartbroken when she saw what had happened. She approached the dead beast slowly and embraced him with her trembling hands. She kissed the ugly face and said, "My beloved beast, I will always love you and remember you forever."

As soon as she said so, she unknowingly broke an evil spell, and her beloved beast awoke, opened his big blue eyes, stood up, and turned into a handsome young prince. They got married and lived happily many years ever after.

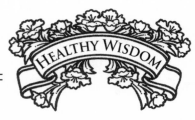

"Trust yourself. You know more than you think you do."

—*Benjamin Spock, MD (1903–1998), known as "Dr. Spock,"*
a U.S. pediatrician and writer

"Laughter is the sun that drives the winter from the human face."

—*Victor Hugo (1802–1885), French novelist, playwright, and poet*

"It is so great to learn every day something new.
The knowledge is the most cheerful thing that everybody wants
to possess, and nobody can take it away from you."

—*Mama*

"No one can make you inferior without your consent."

—*Eleanor Roosevelt (1884–1962), U.S. humanitarian*

"What sunshine is to flowers, smiles are to humanity."

—*Joseph Addison (1672–1719), English writer and statesman*

Chapter 7

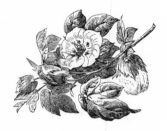

Clever Remedies to Outsmart Headaches

Patience is a flower that does not grow in every garden.

—*English proverb*

FACTS

Estimates indicate that there are more than 45 million headache sufferers in the United States. Only 11 percent of them consult a neurologist for evaluation or treatment. Two-thirds of headache sufferers remain undiagnosed. Headaches account for eight million office visits each year. Most headache sufferers experience two or more concurrent headache types.[22]

As I was browsing in Moscow's Art's Salon, a unique piece of jewelry caught my eye. It was a necklace made in Lithuania, a real masterpiece. Suspended between five layers of delicate silver net was a magnificent piece of golden amber. I slipped it around my neck, fell in love with it, and did not want to take it off. I bought it on the spot and wore it out of the shop. At that time I did not know a lot about the healing properties of amber, but I knew that I felt comfortable wearing it.

Over the years I have learned that this sunny stone helps people feel joyful, inspires love, and stimulates the intellect. Amber necklaces or earrings are said to cleanse the body and mind of negative influences and to purify the air in the room where it rests. When I realized that wearing amber had relieved my headaches, I became extremely interested in this unusual fossilized resin, its history, and Lithuania "the land of amber," where it originated.

The land of amber

Lithuania, a small, scenic country on the Baltic Sea, dates back to the fourteenth century. Its colorful fishing villages, rapid rivers, thousands of crystal blue lakes, and thick green forests draw many visitors.

One summer I stayed in Nida, which is located very close to Klaipeda, one of the biggest ports in Lithuania. Nida, however, is one of the largest and the most beautiful fishing villages on the Curionian Spit, a narrow peninsula separating the Curionian Lagoon from the Baltic Sea. Formed about six thousand years ago, it stretches about 98 kilometers long.

Over many centuries severe, cold northern winds shifted golden sand and created what looks to me like the largest sand dunes in the world. Some of them, like Angiu Kalno and the Urbo Kalno, are approximately a thousand meters high. From the top of the dunes a magnificent view unfolds of the Baltic Sea with its midnight blue waters, as well as the Curionian Lagoon framed by the bright, leafy woods sparkling with morning dew.

Until the fifteenth century coniferous and deciduous forests covered this area, but then people began to cut the trees to build vessels, furniture, and houses. This created a big problem, and Mother Nature reacted in kind when people used some of her natural resources irrationally. The trees' disappearances lead to severe sand shifting and, as a result, the fast-moving sands swallowed 14 villages.

The people undertook the first project to plant new forests in 1825. Fortunately their hard work paid off and the sand stopped shifting. Today the area boasts more than 17,000 acres of pine forests. The range of large sand dunes stretches for about 43 miles and reaches into the Russian territory of Kaliningrad, an area considered the largest amber field in the world. Kaliningrad's famous Amber Museum houses one of the largest collections, consisting of six thousand pieces of jewelry, boxes, and some fragments of the legendary Amber

Room, which was a part of Catherine's the Great summer residence near St. Petersburg, Russia.

When I first arrived in Nida, I was instantly charmed with the tiny, sleepy fishing village of only two thousand residents. It seemed a world apart from civilization, but it was exactly what I wanted. It still held its virgin purity and serene beauty. It was still not touched by modern urbanism and still displayed beautiful wooden architecture.

I had a small room in Nida's resort for youth. At night we would sit in a pine grove near a campfire with local girls and boys and share stories about Lithuania, the land of amber. They told sad and romantic myths and legends about heroic knights and lost love and about the magic of the emerald pine forests. But I remember most the tales they told about amber, the stone of the sun, the tears of the gods, the gold of the sea, and magnificent amber forests and giant trees dripping beads of amber.

I awoke at 6:00 A.M. with a headache and took a walk on the beach. I passed pines that surrounded the hotel like solemn guards. In the still morning hours an elderly Lithuanian woman had already set up a tent with amber souvenirs and handmade jewelry. I looked at what she had to offer, but because of my headache, my eyes were blurry. I rubbed my forehead and the woman said, "Put this amber necklace on and do not remove it for at least two weeks. These stones are the tears of the gods and they will help your headache."

"I had hoped that a walk on the beach, the fresh breeze from the sea, and the smell of the pines would ease it," I replied.

"Oh, it will, but this amber is a powerful healer. You need not pay me any money for this necklace. I am glad to be of service. Go to the shore, take a walk, and forget the headache. Imagine that you may be lucky enough to find pieces of amber. The goddess Jurate still weeps for her lost love, Kastytis, so you may find small amber drops there."

I thanked the old woman and bid her goodbye, and then I walked 10 miles along the shoreline. The sea air was fresh and cool. The old woman's amber necklace warmed my neck. I was focused on finding amber "tears" washed up on the sand by the cold Baltic waters. As I made my way back to the hotel, I realized that my headache was gone. I stopped near the last dune before making the turn to the path in the pine grove and there it was: a dark spark of honey-colored light glistening in the sand. I brushed the sand away and an oval shape like the eye of a mystic animal emerged.

I showed these pieces to a local artist and he made for me a pair of beautiful earrings with silver hooks. I feel energized when I wear them. When I look at them in the mirror, it is as if the amber slowly comes to life, shining like two warm human eyes, as if they are asking us all to plant beautiful flowers and take good care of them, to save a mighty oak tree in a city, a noisy bird in a cage, and a silver star falling down into the sea.

Folk medicine has other remedies for headaches too. Wise elders in Russia told me these ancient myths and superstitions about snakes and their role in curing a headache:

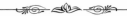

 1. Tie a snakeskin around your head to relieve a headache.

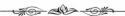

 2. To get rid of headache, "kill it." For example, in Russia people shear a small lock of hair from a person who is suffering from a headache and tie it to a mountain ash tree or to an asp. This "method" was popular in Germany too.

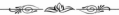

According to Russian folk medicine, however, homemade herbal compresses, nastoykas (infusions), decoctions, ointments, and poultices were most often used to treat headaches. The following suggestions are for external use.

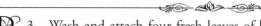

 3. Wash and attach four fresh leaves of burdock to your forehead and your calves. Relax. Or apply leaves of coltsfoot to your forehead to soothe headaches and hot flashes of menopause.

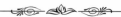

To take control of a headache best,
begin to listen to your body.

*C*ong ago under the midnight blue water of the Baltic Sea stood a magnificent, white amber castle with doors of gold and windows of diamonds. Jurate, the goddess of the sea, lived there.

One day she called a meeting of beautiful maidens, nymphs, and sirens. She told them, "Dear friends, my father Praamzis, the god of the sky, earth, and the sea, gave me these waters of the Baltic Sea to rule. You know that I have never hurt anyone in my life, and we have lived in peace for a long time. But there can be no quiet, happy life anymore. Kastytis, an evil fisherman, takes my innocent servants, my darling fishes, from the water and allows them to die on the shore. I must punish him. I will throw him into the coldest depths of the sea."

The next morning a hundred amber boats took Jurate and her guests in search of the fisherman. The day was bright and sunny and the sea was calm. The trees and flowers were blossoming profusely on the shore, echoing the beauty of the songs sung by the goddess Jurate and her hand-maidens.

The amber vessels sped along until soon they were at the mouth of the river, watching the young, handsome angler empty his net after a good catch. Suddenly he heard the haunting voices of the women. In the center of them stood a statuesque young woman with glistening skin and long, shimmering silver hair. She stood radiant upon a fountain of sea foam, which when struck by sunlight created a sparkling blaze of aurora borealis lights at her feet. She saw Kastytis, who stood entranced on the shore, and she fell in love with him.

"I am Jurate," she said. "I am the goddess of the Baltic Sea and I am immortal. I had come here to punish you for catching my fish, but I will not kill you if you will promise no longer to harm my water kingdom and to pledge to me your love. If you refuse me this, you will die."

The young fisherman knelt before Jurate and promised to love her forever. "From now on I'll meet you every evening on the top of the mountain that I have named after you—Kastytis," said Jurate.

When Praamzis discovered that Jurate had fallen in love with the young human fisherman, he was outraged. He commanded Perkunas, the god of thunder, to toss a lightning bolt into the sea to destroy Jurate's palace. Perkunas killed Jurate and chained Kastytis to a rock at the bottom of the sea.

To this day, whenever there is a storm at sea, the pitiful cries of the young fisherman can be heard as he tosses out honey, orange, brown, and white fragments of amber that wash up with the tide—the remains of Jurate's castle. It is said that lucky beachcombers can still find these stones, created fifty million years ago from the tears of evergreen pines, mourning the sad destiny and lost love of Jurate and Kastytis.

Learn to spot your headache triggers

Researchers tell us that headaches are the most common type of pain that people experience. Headaches come in all different sizes and are caused by many different stimuli. Learn to recognize your headache triggers and symptoms, perhaps by keeping a diary, in which you record the date of your headaches, the length and severity of your headache, foods and fluids you consumed prior to the headache, etc. You will begin to see a pattern that can help you identify which type of headache you experience and help you avoid triggers that might bring a headache on. Of course, if you experience severe headaches that just get worse, see a doctor as soon as possible to determine their cause.

According to the American Council for Headache Education in Mount Royal, New Jersey, emotional stress can trigger or worsen some types of headaches including tension headaches and migraines. To avoid stress-related headaches, work on eliminating as much stress as you can. How? Doctors suggest exercising regularly, getting enough sleep, allowing time for relaxation and hobbies, getting massages, and practicing meditation.

Headache sometimes accompanies diseases of internal organs, poisoning, infections, and nervous and mental disorders. It can also be provoked by poor blood circulation in the brain (migraine), by increase in blood pressure (hypertension), or by a surplus or blood stagnation in the vessels or an accumulation of products in the blood, which can upset the metabolism. It is important to learn to recognize the causes of frequent headaches.

"Tension-type headaches are the most common, affecting upwards of 75 percent of all headache sufferers. Tension-type headaches are typically a steady ache rather than a throbbing one and affect both sides of the head. Some people get tension-type (and migraine) headaches in response to stressful events or a hectic day."[23]

FACTS

Migraine headaches are less common than tension-type headaches. Nevertheless, migraines afflict 25 to 30 million people every year in the United States alone. As many as 6 percent of all men and up to 18 percent of all women experience a migraine attack at some time. This equals about 12 percent of the population as a whole. Roughly three out of four migraine sufferers are female. Usually migraine attacks are occasional, or sometimes as often as once or twice a week, but not daily.[24] By age 15, 15 percent of all teens have experienced a migraine attack. Fifty-eight percent of migraine attacks require some bed rest for a total of 112 million migraine-related bedridden days per year for the U.S. population. Migraine costs to employers from missed days and impaired work function are estimated at $13 billion annually.[25] By age 15, 15

Remember:

The following advice is garnered both from the scientific field and people's medicine, or folk medicine. The treatments may be useful in the treatment of headaches of various origins and character. Any headache treatment must have not only a pain-relieving effect, but it should also help to eliminate the cause of the pain.

If you decide to use these remedies, do so after consulting your doctor or other qualified health-care practitioner. Let your doctor/specialist guide you in the systematic use of these remedies.

percent of all teens have experienced a migraine attack. Fifty-eight percent of migraine attacks require some bed rest for a total of 112 million migraine-related bedridden days per year for the U.S. population. Migraine costs to employers from missed days and impaired work function are estimated at $13 billion annually.[26]

Migraine sufferers say they did not see a doctor about their headache because of misdiagnosis and a belief that their physicians weren't helping them.[27]

Migraine

One of the most common headaches, a migraine, is characterized by sudden pain, often accompanied by blurred vision, dizziness, drowsiness, and loss of energy. Headaches might intensify and may be accompanied by nausea and vomiting, as well as sensitivity to sound and light. A migraine can last from several hours to several days. Some scientists believe migraines are the result of poor blood circulation in the brain. Often they are caused by a short-term spasm of the vessels, which increases pressure and pain. "Migraines are felt on one side of the head by about 60 percent of migraine sufferers, and the pain is typically throbbing in nature."[28]

People who suffer frequent migraines should seek a doctor's advice because severe headaches can be a symptom of serious disease.

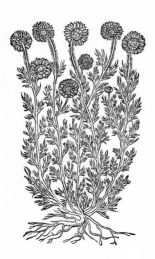

Chamomile, the motherly herb

Look at the night sky full of stars. It looks like a miraculous island of lights. An ancient legend tells us that one night tiny stars dropped from the sky and fell to the earth as chamomile flowers.

Chamomile, because of its rich medicinal properties, is used extensively in many natural remedies throughout this book. The Latin name for chamomile is *Matricaria Chamomilla*. The name is derived from the Latin word *mater*, which means mother. A kind herbal healer for the people, chamomile is like a good nurturing mother and is a favorite, valued folk remedy in Europe, especially in Russia.

$\mathcal{I}$n the mid-nineteenth century chamomile was displayed in a famous St. Petersburg botanical garden as a rare flower—30 years later it grew everywhere in Russia. Chamomile made her way from America to Russia quite easily. As American farmers harvested their fields of grain, small chamomile seeds were collected as well and inadvertently placed into burlap sacks with the grain into the holding compartments of ships. They were "bilkers"—passengers without tickets.

Upon arrival in Russia, the grain was moved by rail. Some sacks were travel worn and ruptured, spilling their contents onto the floors and through cracks where the seeds were sown along the railway. A short time later embankments along the route flourished with the soft, aromatic herb. This is how chamomile seeds passed through several Russian borders undetected and became a permanent flower of my homeland, a staple in our pharmacies, kitchens, and hearts, thousands of miles from America, their native land.

Try the following remedies to ease headache!

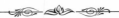

 4. Drink fresh carrot juice.

 5. Administer an enema mixture of herbal laxative such as chamomile, valerian root, horehound, horsetail, or dandelion for relief of occasional constipation and bowel cleansing.

 6. Apply a hot water or vinegar compress to the forehead.

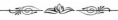

 7. Drink hot Indian tea mixed with Ceylon and lemon.

 8. Drink hot green tea with jasmine.

 9. With both hands, massage your head from your forehead to the base of your skull.

 10. Boil two tablespoons cherries in two cups water for five to seven minutes. Add a pinch of sugar and drink as a hot tea.

 11. Inhale vapors of a mixture of one tablespoon of camphor and one tablespoon of spirits of ammonia. Or try soothing aroma-therapy by inhaling vapors of two to three drops of essential oil of peppermint or lavender added to one cup of water, which has been brought to boiling and removed from heat source.

 12. Drink one glass of spring water on an empty stomach every morning for two to three weeks.

 13. In a small pot combine two teaspoons of peppermint leaves with one cup of boiled water. Steep for three to five minutes, stirring occasionally. Filter and add ½ cup of boiled water. Drink one to three times daily 15 minutes before eating. This tea will keep in the refrigerator for two days.

 14. Ease migraines with contrast baths: alternate about six hot and cold water dips for hands and feet.

 15. Rest your head on a pillow filled with a medicinal herb such as lavender. Try sleeping on it for at least two hours for a luxuriously soothing and simple treatment.

 16. Drink ½ cup fresh cranberry juice.

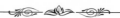

17. Drink one ounce of fresh potato juice.

 18. Make linden tea and drink it hot. It is a good sedative and pain reliever.

 19. Before bed take one tablespoon of sugar or honey and wash it down with one glass of spring water. Do this for several days. This helps a stress headache.

 20. Drink primrose tea.

 21. Place one teaspoon of primrose (roots, leaves, and stems) in a mug. Add boiling water and let steep for 30 minutes. Drink two to four ounces twice daily.

 Note:

Primrose should not be confused with Evening primrose (*Oenothera biennis*). This tea acts as a sedative and has a light soporific effect. However, taken in excess, this tea can cause excitability. Do not exceed recommended dosage.

Chronic headaches

Chronic headaches of nervous origin may occur in the head, temples, or forehead. Some people experience scalp pain, which may indicate oversensitivity. People who suffer from chronic headaches may need rest and/or the following:

 22. Vitamin C, vitamin B complex.

 23. To eliminate or ease nervous headache, try Egg Milk. In a small bowl beat one fresh egg and slowly add 3/4 cup scalded milk. Beat together and drink at once. Follow this simple method every day for 10 days.

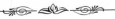

24. With the fingertips apply light pressure to the temples for 10-15 seconds. Release the pressure. Blood will flow into your head to ease the headache

 25. Soak feet to the ankles in hot water for 10 to 15 minutes.

26. Cut a raw potato into thin slices, wrap in two layers of gauze or cheesecloth, and use as a compress on the forehead for 10-15 minutes.

27. When you come home after many hours of working on a computer, you may suffer from what I call brainwork fatigue. To revitalize yourself, try this: Take a warm bath with chamomile. Add five bags of chamomile tea to two cups of boiling water. Steep for 10 minutes, add to bath, and relax in the tub for at least 30 minutes.

28. Ease a sudden headache without special symptoms by adding three drops of glycerin to hot, not boiling, water. Place your elbows in the water until your headache decreases (usually about 20-30 minutes). Add water when necessary to maintain a high temperature.

Headache related to anemia

Because of poor blood circulation, people who suffer from anemia often complain of headaches. You will recognize if anemia is the cause of your pain by several symptoms: forehead becomes cold, pupils dilate, and pulse rate drops. Try this:

29. Tie a cotton kerchief around your head and sit up, elevating your feet. It is important that your feet are the same level as your head. Drink a small cup of strong black coffee or cold raspberry,

strawberry, or chamomile tea. Make sure that you maintain a regular schedule for meals to ensure that you do not become constipated. If constipation occurs, you may find it necessary to cleanse your system with an enema. Afterwards relax with a cold chamomile compress to the forehead.

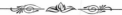

Headache related to flatulence

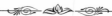

30. Administer an enema of boiled and cooled water (warm or room temperature) or chamomile tea. Then melt in your mouth a cube of refined sugar to which has been added five to seven drops of lavender oil. **Make sure to use unadulterated essential oil of lavendar that does not contain chemicals or perfumes.** Following this, you will begin to feel better.

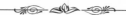

31. Honey tea—**Careful, some people are allergic to honey, particularly the tropical blends of honey.** For those who can eat honey, the following recipe taken two to three times daily can offer some relief from gas. Add one tablespoon of honey and a slice of lemon to a mug of boiling water. Enjoy!

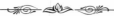

32. No fooling! Soak your socks in water. While still wet, put them on and cover them with a pair of dry socks and a warm blanket. Try this for a few days. It is best to do this before bedtime and keep the wet and dry socks on your feet while you sleep.

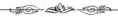

33. Hot, strong black tea with lemon works well when combined with a pinch of peppermint. Black tea helps dilate the blood vessels to ease headaches. I have used this simple healing remedy many times and find that it offers relief. However, I advise you to limit your intake of black tea because it is a stimulant like coffee and may disrupt sleep.

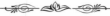

34. In combination with the tea therapy described in #33, you can try this five-minute exercise. Shake your head (gently) two to

three times up and two to three times down. Shake your head two to three times to the right shoulder, then two to three times to the left shoulder. Relax the muscles in your neck, and then turn your head slowly from one side to the other. After you do this exercise several times, your headache may cease. If not, try again in a few minutes.

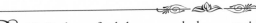

 35. Brew strong Chinese green tea (plain, lemon, lime, orange, or tangerine) with a pinch of mint. Drink one mug.

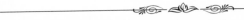

 36. Peel one fresh lemon and place wet side of the peel down on the temples.

 37. Chew a few leaves of feverfew.

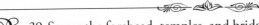

 38. My grandma used a compress of chamomile and strong black tea. Put one teaspoon each of chamomile and black tea in a glass pitcher. Add one cup of boiling water. Let steep for five to seven minutes. Then soak cheesecloth in this liquid, wring it out, and wrap around your head.

39. Smear the forehead, temples, and bridge of nose with the juice of a fresh black radish.

The magic of garlic and onions

Did you know that garlic and onion were used as amulets on the battlefield? In Europe during the Middle Ages soldiers and knights put garlic or onion on their helmets and in their armor. They used iron shields to protect themselves and wore garlic and onions around their necks to defend themselves against the enemy swords and arrows.

Garlic and onion were found in sarcophagi with mummies of Egyptian pharaohs six thousand years ago. In the sixteenth century garlic was used to protect against the Black Death (plague), as an antidote for poisons, and as treatment for tuberculosis and arteriosclerosis.

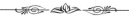

 40. Place wet side of onion slices as compress on forehead.

 41. Mash garlic; put it inside three layers of cheesecloth, and use as a compress on your forehead.

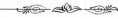 42. Place a washed, fresh geranium (*Gerania odorius*) leaf as a compress on the forehead.

 43. Valerian root, known throughout Europe and particularly in Russia from the Middle Ages, has a pungent smell and a bitter taste. This unique healer calms nerves and reduces the pressure of a headache. It promotes digestion, warms the alimentary canal, and eases mild depression and intestinal diseases.

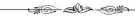

Nastoykas

Right or wrong, and definitely contrary to the doctrines of Western medicine that promotes drinking at least eight eight-ounce glasses of water daily and limiting alcohol intake, my grandpa rarely drank water. Instead he drank his own homemade wine which he called "Sunny Beams." Curiously he never was drunk, he never was sick, and he lived to be 89. After he died, doctors told us that his blood vessels were "as clean as an 18-year-old's."

Nastoyka is Russian for a specially prepared liquor or infusion. The following are some familiar nastoykas used by my family for years to treat nervous tension (especially anxiety and insomnia), to strengthen the heart, to improve digestion, and sometimes to reduce high blood pressure.

Valerian Nastoyka

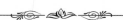

 44. Cut small pieces of valerian root (one tablespoon) or use 10–15 500-mg powdered valerian capsules. Add five tablespoons of 70-percent vodka. Store in a warm place for one week, and shake it occasionally. Pass the liquid through a sieve and the nastoyka is ready to use. Take about 15 drops a day as a sedating brew for sleeplessness and anxiety.

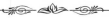

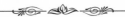

45. Cut valerian root (or 10–15 capsules) into small pieces to equal one tablespoon. Add four tablespoons of 70-percent vodka. Store for four days. Then add one teaspoon of lemon juice or three drops of peppermint water available from pharmacies to disguise the flavor. Let steep for an additional three days. Pass the liquid through a sieve. You will have a solution with a yellow tint. Take 10 drops twice daily as a sedative or for insomnia.

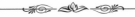

46. Add two tablespoons (about 20 capsules) of ground valerian root to a bath. This is an excellent remedy for nervousness, sleepless-ness, headaches, stomach pains, and spasms of the uterus.

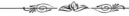

47. Valerian root in 470–500 mg capsules is effective for easing symptoms of pneumonia, migraine, and scarlet fever. Take two to three capsules three to four times daily with eight ounces of water or three to four capsules 30 minutes before bedtime.

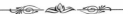

48. Mince two tablespoons of valerian root and place in a mug. Add one glass of cold water. Let steep for six to eight hours. Filter. Take one tablespoon three times daily as a sedative or for insomnia.

Caution:

Valerian enhances the action of sleep-inducing drugs. Avoid it if taking this type of medication. Take Valerian for only two to three weeks without a break as continual use may lead to palpitations and headaches.

Don't confuse Valerian (*Valeriana officinalis*) with red "American" valerian (*Centranthus rubber*), a garden plant, which has no medicinal properties.

It is known that St. John's Wort takes its name from the Knights of St. John of Jerusalem, who used this plant to treat wounds of the injured on Crusade battlefields. In Russia, St. John's Wort is called a healer of 99 diseases. It is used extensively in many herbal concoctions because of its ability to soothe a wide range of ailments, such as inflamma-tions and injuries, jaundice, hysteria, depression, anxiety, and irritability, espe-cially during menopause. Some plants, such as raspberries, lose their effectiveness in dried form, but St. John's Wort is an effective healer in fresh or dried form.

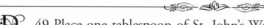

 49. Place one tablespoon of St. John's Wort in a mug. Add boiling water. Leave to infuse for 15 minutes. Filter and drink three tablespoons three times a day for anxiety, emotional upsets, and nervous tension.

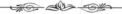

Elecampane was one of the most important herbs to the Romans and Greeks. By the nineteenth century it was widely used for stubborn coughs and congestion, colds, bronchitis, neuralgia, and skin problems. In Russia elecampane root is called the "nine powers herb." It is used as a tonic for weakness following colds and to treat headaches provoked by upper respiratory problems.

 50. Slice thinly a small elecampane root. Boil one teaspoon for 15 minutes in one cup water. Cool, filter, and drink three tablespoons three times daily.

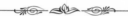

 51. Place one tablespoon dried elder flowers in eight ounces boiling water and steep for 20 minutes. Filter and add one teaspoon honey. Drink two ounces three or four times daily 15 minutes before eating. This tea is best prepared fresh each time you use it.

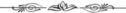

 52. If you suffer from chronic headaches that occur monthly or weekly, try this simple remedy: Juice a potato and drink two ounces two to three times daily.

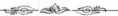

 53. When you are overtired, your "head is swimming," and you feel giddy from exhaustion, try this: Mix 1½ tablespoons hawthorn berries with 1½ tablespoons hawthorn flowers. Add 24 ounces boiling water and steep for two hours in a warm place. Filter and take one tablespoon three times daily 30 minutes before eating.

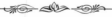

54. Ginseng helps fight fatigue and headache. Cut one tablespoon ginseng root into small pieces and place in a mug with four ounces Port wine or cognac. Let steep five to seven days. Take 15 drops twice daily.

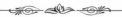

Vegetables were extremely important as "food therapy" while I was growing up in southeastern Europe. Every evening our family dinner began with a large porcelain bowl brimming with seasonal vegetables from our own garden. In summer, bright red tomatoes and white and green onions would always find their way to the salad bowl to be dressed with olive oil, sunflower oil, or sometimes sour cream. After the salad bowl was placed on the table and just before the family would gather for dinner, Grandma added the freshly harvested dill that I had previously gathered from a large patch in the garden. This simple daily ritual helped to maintain the freshness and aroma of the dill. Grandma's fresh-baked and fragrant rye bread was always nearby.

We rarely ate meat. Instead our menu sometimes consisted of stuffed cabbage (golubtsi), zucchini, green and red bell peppers, mashed potatoes, beans and eggplant, homemade fruit drinks and fresh fruits, herbal teas, or compotes.

Here are some natural vegetable remedies for headaches.

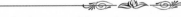

 55. Apply fresh, raw cabbage leaves to the forehead for 10-15 minutes.

 56. Eat a bowl of fresh strawberries.

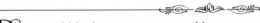

 57. Add boiling water to one tablespoon sweet clover flowers in a mug. Steep for 30 minutes. Filter and drink four ounces three times daily.

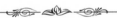

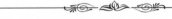 58. In a bowl add one pint of boiling water to one tablespoon oregano. Cover bowl with a plate and thick towel and steep for 30 minutes. Sweeten with honey, filter, and drink 4–16 ounces (depending on the severity of the headache) three times a day. **Pregnant women should not use this remedy.**

 59. In Russia the herb lemon balm is called melissa, lemon balm, or lemon mint. Place 1½ tablespoons of lemon balm in a mug with boiling water. Cover with a thick towel and steep for 30 minutes.

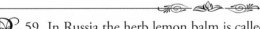

Filter and drink one to two tablespoons five or six times daily. Lemon balm is a natural sedative that treats headache, sleeplessness, stress, heart pains, palpitation (tachycardia), anemia, colic, "swimming head," and inflamed bowels.

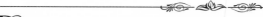

 60. Juice fresh black currants and drink two ounces three times a day for chronic headaches. Do this for at least one week and the headaches should cease.

 61. Prepare calendula tincture. Calendula is ***not bur marigold, which is toxic if taken internally.*** To one ounce of calendula add three ounces vodka and steep for two weeks. Take 20–30 drops three times a day. Your headaches should disappear, your sleep should improve, and your efficiency should increase. Calendula tincture rapidly quells inflammation, speeds the regeneration of tissues, and aids in healing wounds.

 62. Peppermint oil rubbed on the forehead, temples, and neck and behind the ears eases headaches related to colds and sinus congestion.

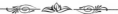

Headaches provoked by colds

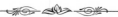

 63. Rub forehead and temples with the grated rind of a lemon.

 64. Add a pinch of cinnamon to one pint of hot water and steep for 30 minutes. Add sugar or honey. Take two tablespoons every hour.

 65. Add ½ teaspoon cinnamon to one tablespoon hot water. Steep for 30 minutes. Use as a lotion to rub on the temples.

 66. To alter the fragrance of cinnamon, add to it one drop of mint or lavender oil.

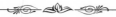

67. To one quart of boiling water, add eight ounces freshly mashed hawthorn berries. Add sugar or honey and steep for 30 minutes. Drink two mugs before bed to ease headache and provide sound sleep.

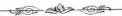

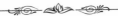 68. To one tablespoon thyme (leaves and flowers) add eight ounces boiling water. Steep for 10 minutes. Drink two ounces three times a day.

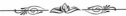 69. People who suffer from hypertension very often have headaches because of high blood pressure. A simple remedy is to add to 24 ounces of boiling water the dried peel of two red onions. Leave to infuse for one hour. Drink one glass three times a day one hour before eating.

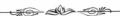 70. People's medicine in Russia and other European countries tell us that the best way to treat headaches and pain in the hands is by listening to the gentle, healing tinkling of a bell.

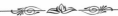

I suffered with chronic headaches for a period in my life when I was not eating at the right times. I worked many hours and was under a tremendous amount of stress. I got rid of these painful and bothersome headaches for a long time.

How I believe I got rid of them and how I keep them at bay today may sound a bit unusual, but I believe it is true. I wear Baltic amber around my neck. When I was plagued by those terrible, throbbing headaches, I wore my favorite stone for two weeks 24 hours a day. The recurring headaches disappeared. No kidding!

Since ancient times in various parts of the world, amber has been called, among other things, tears of the gods, gold of the North, gold of the sea, and stones of the sun. It is said to clean the environment in which it rests. It is believed to be a symbol of renewal in troubled marriages and a generator of new love relationships. It is also said to stimulate the intellect, clear thinking, activate unconditional love in people, and open the crown chakra.

Generation after generation searched for the origin of the discovery of amber, and it is said that the first sunny stone was found near the Sunset (Baltic) Sea. Sometime around the fifteenth century amber began to make itself known. In the eighteenth century Swedish scientist C. Linnaeus (1707–1778) was the first to indicate that amber has a natural origin. Later in the nineteenth century Michael Lomonosov, a prominent Russian scientist, confirmed his theory. In 1812 a rare amber stone was found which contained a small tree twig. This find proved the theory that amber is not just a fossilized resin as many sources cite today, but it is the resin that turned into amber because of a chemical process going on for centuries, the influence and interaction of the air and water on the resin, and then "hiding" many years under ground until the stone was found in the thick, green forest.

These forests stretched widely around the Baltic Sea many centuries ago. Some believe that these forests started near the small town of Nida in Lithuania and then reached the Bornholm Island in Denmark in the west and came to Tallinn (Estonia) and Stockholm (Sweden) in the north.

Many times while traveling in the Baltic States, I saw these huge trees, resinous and aromatic near crystal-clear blue rivers that carried amber stones to other rivers, lakes, and seas through the centuries. This natural waterway brought amber to England and Ukraine, but amber's favorite destination seemed to be the Kaliningrad region in Russia. The small town of Yantarny (amber is *yantar* in Russian) once held the title of the biggest amber field in the world.

In ancient times, amber was worth its weight in gold. The demand for it spread throughout many countries. Caravans carried it from the Baltic region to Rome. Stone Age people wore amber for adornment and as a talisman to fend off evil spirits and disease. Long ago Native Americans discovered amber's magic and it became a sacred stone for them. They used it in rituals to manifest desires into reality.

Remember:

Baltic amber has the highest healing power during the first hours of a new moon.

Amber needs a day off. Give your necklace, ring, earrings, or bracelet a rest at the end of each month—preferably on the night before a new moon.

Here's how:
Soak the amber overnight in a crystal bowl filled with water and a pinch of sea salt. The next morning remove the stones from the bowl, wrap in a flax napkin, and dry outside in the sun.

Many stories, myths, and legends about amber are still told by people in the Baltic States, Poland, Romania, Scandinavian countries, Czechoslovakia, and other countries where the sunny gold stone is found.

I feel that it is important for me to wear amber from the Baltic Sea. I also have amber necklaces from India and Israel, but my Baltic amber resonates with me above all and is my personal healer. I feel comfortable with this stone. It provides me with solar and healing energy to combat my headaches.

Baltic amber is the fossilized resin or sap of various ancient trees, specifically the pine tree (*Pinus succinifera*), and was formed during the Eocene period about 50 million years ago. It is found in many locations in the world. Baltic amber takes a higher polish than other ambers and is generally considered the finest in the world. It ranges in color from yellow to light brown and the clarity varies from transparent to opaque. While not the oldest fossilized resin, Baltic amber has the longest historical record of use over many centuries.

For ages amber has been considered folk medicine—a healing stone—able to draw disease out from the human body and ease emotional torment. The medicinal and magnetic influence of honey, red, and brown amber increases if insects and other foreign matter are trapped inside the stone.

Some years ago a guide in Kaliningrad's Amber Museum told me the following story.

An old man strolling along the shore of the Baltic Sea found a huge, rare piece of amber and took it to a castle in Konigsberg. The stone sparkled with golden light and was distinct because it displayed a shiny silver snake coiled inside. Out of curiosity the monks began to pass it among themselves. When the fourth monk took the stone, he turned it upside down. The fifth monk, who was waiting patiently to touch it, exclaimed, "Look, brothers, the snake is now alive!"

"This is a miracle!" the sixth monk said.

"Don't pass this stone to me," said the seventh monk. "Perhaps it is touched by evil."

They buried the stone in a secret spot and retrieved it only when the French went to war with the monks' people, the Prussians. The monks

---

showed their treasure to the French knights, who were amused with the amber containing the coiled silver snake. It wasn't long before news of the miraculous find reached the Pope at the Vatican, who sent messengers to bring the stone to Rome. Meanwhile several French knights wanted to buy the stone, but the monks refused to sell it. They believed the ancient stone was priceless. It could have originated in a primeval forest somewhere in the region of the Baltic (Sunset) Sea and may have lay buried in the ground from the time dinosaurs roamed the earth. But when the French knights persistently offered their glistening gold bars to trade for the stone, the poor monks were lured by the sight of them and sold the amber to the richest French knight before the Pope's messengers arrived.

The stone became an object of worship for the knight who purchased it. He placed the amber on a big table, surrounded by kettles and mirrors that reflected multicolored jewels. The knight became obsessed with watching the snake and could not eat or sleep. He just gazed at the magic stone, which had won his heart and soul.

One evening, as soon as the knight closed his eyes, the amber turned into a slumberous witch. The flames flared under the kettles around the stone. As some mysterious force stoked the fire, the flames grew intense and melted the amber into honey. At once the snake slithered out.

The knight slept soundly as the snake slid silently down the knight's neck and struck him fast near his heart. Still the knight dreamt uninterruptedly of his amber. In the morning his fellow crusaders found him dead. Nearby sat the shining amber with the silver snake inside. The horrified monks buried the stone and marked the site with a warning to others.

The monks mourned the death of the French knight, but the Prussian knights engraved the image of a snake on their bronze belt buckles to commemorate the snake that killed their enemy. The image became a talisman to protect them on the battlefield.

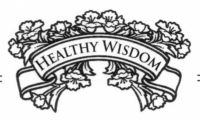

Words are the Physicians.

—*Aeschylus (525-456 B.C.), Greek dramatist*

You can't jump over your own head.

—*Russian proverb*

I take a sun bath and listen to the hours, formulating and disintegrating under the pines, and smell the resiny hardihood of the high-noon hours.

—*Zelda Fitzgerald (1900–1948), American writer*

How far that little candle throws his beams!
So shines a good deed in a naughty world.

—*William Shakespeare (1564–1616), English playwright and poet*

And that was another gap between us. Between all men and all insects.
We humans, saddled for a lifetime with virtually the same body,
naturally find it difficult to imagine a life in which you can,
at a single stroke, outside a fairy tale, just by splitting your skin
and stepping out, change into something utterly different.

—*Colin Fletcher (b.1922), Welsh hiker and writer*

The sea, once it casts its spell, holds one in its net of wonder forever.

—*JacquesYves Cousteau (1910–1997), French marine explorer*

Chapter 8

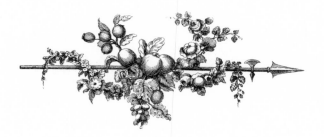

Sleeping Beauty

Life is long, if you know how to use it.

—*Seneca (4 B.C.–A.D. 65), Roman philosopher*

FACTS

Studies estimate that about one-third of American adults experience some insomnia each year, and between 10 and 20 percent suffer severe sleeplessness. European studies suggest similar rates. A recent survey conducted by the national Sleep Foundation reported even worse statistics on sleeplessness in the United States: 1) only 35 percent of American adults reported sleeping eight hours or more per night during the work week; 2) 56 percent had one or more symptoms of insomnia a few nights a week or more; 3) 60 percent of children, particularly teenagers, complained of being tired during the day; 4) over half of the elderly took an hour's nap during the work week and nearly half of 18- to 29-year-olds napped.[29]

According to statistics, millions of people suffer from sleeplessness. Many of them would be delighted to claim that they occasionally experienced a restful sleep for an adequate length of time. It seems that a sound sleep happens more frequently in fairy tales than in real life.

Like nearly everyone, perhaps you too have had trouble sleeping at one time or another. Simply put, if we do not get enough rest, our overall health is at stake. If you suffer from insomnia or toss and turn restlessly in your sleep, your nerves and cells never get the relaxation and rejuvenation they need to function properly. The result may be fatigue, high blood pressure or low blood pressure, and diseases of the nervous system.

Ruslan and Ludmila

A great feast was held in the halls of Svietosar, the Duke of Kiev. This feast was in honor of his daughter, Ludmila. Three suitors were there to vie for her hand: Ruslan the knight; Ratmir the poet; and Farlaf, a warrior.

When the festivities were at their height, a huge thunderclap boomed, followed by darkness, during which Ludmila mysteriously disappeared. Svietosar was distraught and promised his daughter's hand to the suitor who could find her and bring her home.

Ruslan learned from Finn, a sorcerer, that Ludmila had been abducted by the evil dwarf Chernomor, who had magical powers and soared through the sky with his long white beard flowing around him. Ruslan was also warned about the witch Naina, who was Farlaf's ally.

While Ruslan sought advice from Finn, Farlaf went to Naina for help. She told Farlaf to allow Ruslan to go through all the trials necessary to find Ludmila and then to kidnap her from Ruslan.

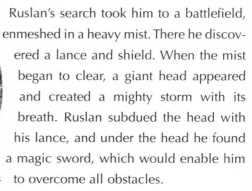

Ruslan's search took him to a battlefield, enmeshed in a heavy mist. There he discovered a lance and shield. When the mist began to clear, a giant head appeared and created a mighty storm with its breath. Ruslan subdued the head with his lance, and under the head he found a magic sword, which would enable him to overcome all obstacles.

Meanwhile, although Ludmila was held captive in Chernomor's castle, she was allowed to walk freely in the beautiful garden behind the tall walls which surrounded the castle. Here she found herself in the midst of majestic trees and a profusion of blossoming flowers, plants, and fragrant herbs. Magnificent peacocks and gentle deer walked beside her. Multicolored birds sang sweet songs from their treetop perches.

But Ludmila was unhappy and could not be consoled by the beauty around her. She feared that she would never be rescued from the evil dwarf Chernomor and returned to her home.

Meanwhile Ruslan rode straight to Chernomor's castle. When he arrived, Chernomor forced Ludmila into a sound sleep and then went to meet the brave knight in battle. With the magic sword Ruslan won the fight with Chernomor. Victorious, he carried Ludmila away even though she was deep into sleep. He despaired because he could not awaken her.

Ruslan returned to Finn to learn how to awaken Ludmila. Finn gave Ruslan a fine ring with magical properties, and with the aid of this ring, he broke Chernomor's spell. Ludmila opened her big blue eyes, sighed, and smiled. Stretching her graceful, long legs, she inquired, "Oh, how long have I slept?"

Just then Farlaf appeared and tried to kidnap Ludmila, but Ruslan vanquished him with his magic sword. That evening Ratmir, the poet, snuck behind Ludmila's tent and tried to lure her outside with his love poems. However she was so tired from her ordeal that she did not respond.

The next day the knight returned Ludmila to her father's palace, where they were greeted with great joy. Ruslan and Ludmila were married amid great festivities and lived together happily for many years.

Experts define sleeplessness or insomnia as sleep disturbance, when one has difficulty falling asleep and/or staying asleep. Some believe, erroneously, that this happens only to elderly people who seem to sleep shorter periods of time than the young. In fact, the luxury of a sound sleep is greatly influenced by the type of lifestyle we lead. No matter what age we are, we might experience several interruptions in our sleep during the night. And then it might take us an hour or more to fall asleep again.

In some cases sleep can be prolonged but still be insufficient. It can be annoying when we would like to sleep, but we cannot in spite of being exhausted. We may complain about lying awake for hours without being able to fall asleep. We may awaken and recount and dwell on the problems in our lives, which often grow in magnitude at the daunting hour of 3:00 A.M. Tensions and pressures accrued during our everyday routines, including demands at the workplace and the negative impact they have on us, can interrupt our sleep and cause depression.

Experts usually classify various modes of sleep into three categories: 1) superficial, when a person can be easily awaked by even a small noise; 2) a deep sleep, bringing satisfaction and rest; and 3) a sleep accompanied by good and bad dreams. When people suffer insomnia, the duration of deep sleep decreases at the expense of a superficial sleep. These changes lead to some problems in the morning. When a person feels tired and jaded, his memory, concentration, and efficiency suffer. In addition, even at the beginning of a new day he may experience headaches and weakness.

Causes of insomnia vary

Even a healthy person can suffer from sleeplessness. Fatigue and irritation inhibit reflexes in the brain's cortex. Any stress can attack the sensitive nervous system and disrupt a good night's sleep. Some people also experience insomnia when they are sick with colds and fever or have poor blood circulation or respiratory problems.

All these conditions prompt the sleepless to get fast treatment, and many reach right for a sleeping pill, which is counterproductive and dangerous. Fast-acting tranquilizers are enemies to the body. Too many people think the sleeping pill is the answer to their problems. On the contrary, they can promote a dependency on them and the consumer may find that he cannot function normally without them—or with them. At this stage the consumer is addicted. Chemical addiction destroys the body's ability to react in a natural way and, left untreated, can eventually lead to death.

The treatment for insomnia depends on the causes that provoke it. Try to discover your triggers and eliminate them. Perhaps you habitually drink alcohol at lunch or at dinnertime or you try to boost your energy, drinking strong black coffee several times a day. Try the following instead. Healthy people are usually able to restore their sleep in 10–14 days without the use of sleeping pills.

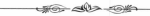

 1. Replace alcohol or coffee with a glass of carrot, tomato, orange, apple, or grape juice. Become accustomed to a new taste. You'll be happy to see that this simple change in your habits can help you to sleep soundly throughout the night.

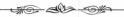

 2. People with sensitive nervous systems should take a walk in the fresh air before bedtime and/or take a warm, calming bath. If not a bath, try a cold shower.

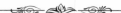

A woman in Kazakhstan created a method of treatment with cold water to cure herself when she got very sick. Then she offered her water treatment technique to her husband, two daughters, and grandchildren. When she was sure that it helped those who tried it, she opened several schools for adults and children, training them in a cold water self-cure technique. You can do it yourself following these simple steps.

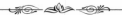

 3. Take a cold shower or swim in a pool with cold water each morning.

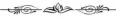

 4. Apply a cold pack (kept in the freezer) to the back of the head or neck before bedtime.

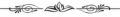

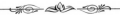

 5. Massage your body in a circular motion with a natural bristle brush to help induce a good night's sleep.

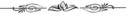

Massage will stimulate blood circulation and drive blood to the external areas of the body. Sleeplessness is often caused by an accumulation of too much blood in the brain. The brain is always at work, 24 hours a day. The mind is always busy, and very often we are under stress, so we need a fair balance between day and night, which requires a deep, sound sleep to preserve our health and energy.

To begin, get familiar with simple folk remedies, which are preventive measures for healthy people with a sensitive nervous system, who are prone to developing insomnia.

 6. Try going to sleep and waking at the same hour each day. You will benefit from a routine biological rhythm. It is important to reach a balance.

Since prevention is better than cure, take good care of your nervous system and heart, which works very hard, constantly pumping blood to your brain and all other internal organs. Many centuries ago King Solomon wisely advised people to take care of their hearts more than anything else. He made a good point by saying that "out of the heart shall flow springs of living water," referring to the Holy Spirit (John 7:38).

In Russia and northern European countries, such as Norway, Sweden, the Netherlands, Finland, and Denmark, sauna baths are very popular. These beneficial treatments are now practiced in many other countries around the world. You'll read more about them in the chapter, "Dialogue with the Trees of Strength and Everlasting Life."

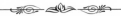

 7. People have enjoyed sauna baths for centuries. After these baths (*banya*), some people, especially in Russia, plunge into icy water or walk barefoot or roll in the freshly fallen snow.

These simple procedures are proven to build the body's resistance to illness and drive the blood from the brain to be distributed equally throughout internal organs and the skin. This procedure promotes a healthy, restful sleep. You'll read more about calming bath remedies later in this chapter. The following are simple folk remedies that have proven successful for many years. Try them and enjoy the sleep of the just.

 8. Drink a cup of warm water or milk sweetened with a little honey or sugar before bedtime.

 9. Drink a cup of "Tranquility" tea. Place one tablespoon minced valerian root in a cup and add boiling water. Steep for 20 minutes. Filter and drink.

10. Add one tablespoon valerian root to eight ounces boiling water. Continue to boil for 15 minutes. Steep for 10 minutes. Filter and take one tablespoon twice daily.

 11. Cold valerian drink. Dice one tablespoon valerian root. Add one cup cold boiled water. Steep for 24 hours. Take five to six teaspoons a day.

 12. Take a 30-minute walk outside before bedtime.

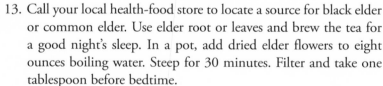 13. Call your local health-food store to locate a source for black elder or common elder. Use elder root or leaves and brew the tea for a good night's sleep. In a pot, add dried elder flowers to eight ounces boiling water. Steep for 30 minutes. Filter and take one tablespoon before bedtime.

In the chapter "Stop Sneezes and Sniffles and Stifle a Cold" I wrote about the black elder plant as a "treasure chest" of the green pharmacy. If you are awake right now and cannot sleep, perhaps you would like to read the funny superstitions about this great plant.

- In the seventeenth century there was a belief that if a small boy got scratched by an elder branch, he stopped growing.

- Lightning never hits the elder, so some people plant it near their houses for protection.

- If you want to get rid of a wart, rub it with a green branch of elder. Then bury the branch in the ground to rot—the wart will disappear.

- If a horseman carries two small branches of elder in his pocket, he will never rub a sore on his horse's back, no matter how fast he gallops. Even today some horsemen carry the twigs of elder in their pockets during horse races.

- Cut a piece of elder branch between two "joints," where the sunlight has never fallen and hang around the neck of an epileptic to treat his condition. This treatment was popular in Europe in the seventeenth century.

- Elder was considered an effective healer in many European countries. Various beliefs surrounding this plant created legends, such as that the cross on which Jesus Christ was crucified was made of elder, and traitor Judas hanged himself on the elder tree too. Contrary to British beliefs, Russian legends tell that the cross on which Jesus was crucified was made from the cypress, but Judas hanged himself on the asp.

- Slavic people bent young shoots of elder from the tree to the ground and held them there with stones. A sick person with fever was to crawl three times under the arch of the elder's branches and say, "I cut out my sickness with these three shoots." The same ceremony was performed in England as well, but instead of the elder, they used the sprouts of an oak or an asp.

- According to Russian folk beliefs, the elder possessed a magic. The elder's cane saved and defended a traveler from wicked people and dangerous animals.

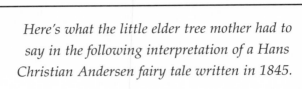

hat was no fairy tale," said the little elder tree mother, "but now it comes!" Real life furnishes us with subjects for the most wonderful fairy tales; for otherwise my beautiful elder bush could not have grown forth from a teapot.

She took the little boy from his bed and placed him on her bosom; the elder branches, full of blossoms, closed over them. It was as if they sat in a thick, leafy bower which flew with them through the air; it was beautiful beyond all description. Suddenly the elder tree mother became a charming young girl with a green dress covered with white blossoms, just as the elder tree mother had worn; she wore an elder blossom on her bosom, and a wreath of the same flowers was wound round her curly golden hair. Her eyes were large and sky blue. Those who gazed into them were mesmerized. She and the boy kissed each other, and then they became the same age and felt the same joys.

They walked about hand-in-hand and then the little girl seized the boy round the waist, and they flew far into the country. It was spring and it became summer, it was autumn and it became winter, and thousands of pictures reflected themselves in the boy's eyes and heart and the little girl always sang, "You will never forget that!" During their flight the elder tree smelled so sweet for the flowers fixed on the little girl's bosom lay against the little boy's face as he rested his head against her and slept soundly throughout the flight.

Try the benefits of herbs for sleep, using the following remedies:

 14. Combine one teaspoon of minced elecampane root and one cup cold water. Steep for 10 hours. Filter and drink two ounces four times daily 30 minutes before eating.

 15. Combine 1½ ounces dried dill or dill seeds with one pint of Port wine or grape juice. Cook seeds in wine over a low heat for 10 minutes. Drink one wine glass before bedtime.

Two ancient Russian remedies

 16. Place a birch broom under your pillow. This plant will induce sleep.

 17. Place under your pillow a handful of hops. You'll have a sound sleep in a state of natural "intoxication."

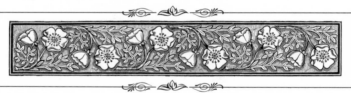

 18. Drink ⅓ glass Cabernet Sauvignon or Chardonnay, which act as natural sleeping remedies and stimulate sleep.

To combat headaches and sleeplessness, my Grandma used the remedies and recipes previously described and also an unusual, but proven environmental alteration, using black sheets. This method has offered excellent results even for those who have suffered for months with sleeplessness and nightmares.

Before bedtime she would cover a window in her bedroom with black cotton fabric. When I asked her why, she said that the black fabric reminded her of the night sky and it helped her to get a quiet sleep.

As a student at Moscow University, I observed the same ritual in the home of a famous Russian poet. She was widely recognized during the 1970s along with other celebrated poets in Russia, including Andrey Voznesensky and

Eugene Evtushenko. Her poems, rich with strong emotions and philosophies, entertained hundreds of readers.

During one period in her life, she nearly suffered a nervous breakdown due to sleep deprivation.

It was in summer when I, then a reporter, set out to interview her for an article for a local newspaper. I visited her in her country home, a *dacha* set in Peredelkino, a small village near Moscow nestled in a beautiful northern forest where some of the most renowned poets and writers in Russia wrote their most inspiring works. In fact, it was there that Boris Pasternak wrote his classic novel, *Doctor Zhivago*.

"*Zdravstvuy!*" she said, bidding me hello as she opened the door. In a less enthusiastic tone she told me she was not feeling well, but to please come into her bedroom.

Once in the room she returned to her bed, and I, surprised by the room's ominous appearance, asked her why her sheets, pillows, comforter, and even her nightgown were made of black silky satin.

"The color black soothes my mind and gives me unbelievable, amazing tranquility; rapt attention to my poems; and sound sleep," she explained, "so I can completely relax from my everyday thoughts, problems and brainwash."

We continued our conversation for a couple of hours and at the end I was not overexcited from having just interviewed a great talent in Russian poetry. Instead I began to feel sleepy. The black color around me had become dominant in my mind.

I later learned that experiments have shown that people who have tried many remedies for sleeplessness to no avail have found rest from the extensive use of the color black or navy in their bedrooms. Try this to get a sound sleep:

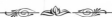

 19. Make your bed in thin black or navy fine satin fabric: sheets, pillowcase, comforter, and nightgown or pajamas. If you are really adventurous, you can even paint your walls black and add shimmering silver stars.

 20. Rub your temples with lavender oil before you go to sleep.

 21. Pour five drops of pure lavender oil into a cube of sugar. Let it melt in your mouth before bedtime.

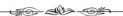

 22. Place ½ ounce celery stalk (Apium graveolens) in a glass jar. Add one quart of cold boiled water for eight hours, then filter. Take one teaspoon three times a day to help prolong your sleep.

 23. Crush two tablespoons dried red hawthorn berries and place in a glass jar. Add 1½ cups of boiling water. Steep for 30 minutes. Take the mixture three times daily 30 minutes before a meal. It is a helpful treatment for insomnia for those with heart disease.

 24. Place one tablespoon oats in a large jar. Add two cups of cold boiled or spring water and cover overnight. Next morning cook for five minutes. Drink it as a tea any time for a better sleep.

 25. Cook eight ounces oats and five cups cold boiled or spring water in an enamel pot until volume is reduced by half. Filter, add four teaspoons of honey, and cook for an additional 30 minutes. Drink two to three times daily. The tea is a good natural calmative/sedative.

 26. Place two tablespoons crushed turnip roots in an enamel pot. Add one cup water and cook 15 minutes. Drink ¼ cup four times daily or one glass before bedtime.

 27. Wild lettuce usually is referred to as the bitter cousin of common garden lettuce. It has been known for its mild sedative and painkilling effects since Greek and Roman times. Place two teaspoons of crushed, dried leaves of wild lettuce in a mug and add one cup of boiling water. Steep for 10 minutes, filter and drink ½ cup before bed. It induces sound sleep, relieves pain and can ease nervousness and muscle spasms. Do not drive or operate machinery when taking this infusion.

 28. Put two teaspoons honey and one teaspoon apple vinegar in a mug. Mix and take at bedtime. This usually induces sleep within 30 minutes. If you are overtired and feel weak and you wake up in the middle of the night, repeat the same. Honey itself stimulates sleep. It becomes more effective in combination with apple cider.

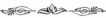

Remedies treating insomnia of nervous origin, including headache, neurasthenia, or neurosis

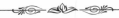

29. Boil one tablespoon red elderberries in one cup water for 15 minutes. Steep for 20 minutes. Filter and take twice a day.

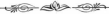

30. Make a nastoyka (infusion) from the passionflower *(Passiflora incarnata)*. Place one tablespoon of crushed, dried leaves of Passionflower in a mug and add one cup of boiling water. Steep for 10 minutes, strain and drink ½ mug before going to bed. Do not drive or operate machinery, because the nastoyka acts as a sedative. The fresh or dried whole plant is used effectively as an herbal medicine to treat anxiety and insomnia.

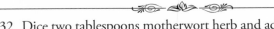

31. Dice two teaspoons motherwort herb *(Leonurus cardiaca)* and add one cup boiled or spring water. Steep for eight hours. Use it all within one day.

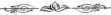

32. Dice two tablespoons motherwort herb and add 2½ cups boiling water. Steep for two hours. Drink ½ cup four times a day before meals. It is a good calming and sedative natural medicine.

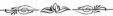

33. Blend one teaspoon peppermint, one teaspoon motherwort, one teaspoon valerian root, and two teaspoons hops. Place one table-spoon of herbal mixture in an enamel cup. Add one cup of boiling water. Place this cup in a pot with boiling water for 15 minutes for a steaming water bath. Cool and filter. Take ½ cup two times a day for insomnia, irritation, and nervous excitement.

34. Place two tablespoons lemon balm in two cups boiling water. Steep until cooled. Take all during the day in equal portions. It acts as a calming sedative.

35. Mix one teaspoon strobiles (dried female flowers in leafy cone-like catkins) of hops and one teaspoon chopped valerian root. Add one tablespoon of the mixture to one cup boiling water. Let it steep for 15 minutes. Take ½ cup only before bedtime for insomnia.

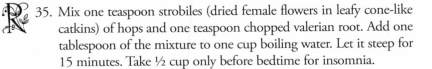

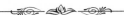

36. Mix five teaspoons thyme, four teaspoons wild marjoram, five teaspoons motherwort, four teaspoons valerian root, and one teaspoon yellow sweet clover/sweet Lucerne (Melilotus officinalis). Add two tablespoons of the mixture to one pint boiling water. Steep for two hours. Drink ½ cup three times daily before a meal as a calming remedy.

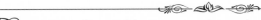

37. Mix three tablespoons each motherwort and valerian root and two tablespoons lemon balm. Add one tablespoon of the mixture to 1½ cups boiling water. Steep for two hours. Filter and drink ½ cup three times daily before a meal. It is helpful for insomnia, neurosis, and erratic heartbeat as a calming and sedating substance.

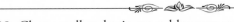

38. Chop small and mix one tablespoon each of lemon balm, motherwort, strobiles of hops, valerian root, wild marjoram, peppermint, young leafy twigs of mistletoe (*Viscum album*). Put one tablespoon of the mixture in a cup and add 1 cup boiling water. Steep for 30 minutes. Filter and drink ½ cup twice a day, in the morning and in the evening, 30 minutes before a meal.

Caution:

Never use mistletoe berries, which are toxic. Avoid using mistletoe leaves during pregnancy.

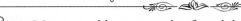

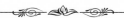

39. Mix one tablespoon each of strobiles of hops, rosemary, peppermint, St. John's Wort, lemon balm, and valerian root. To two tablespoons of this mixture add one cup boiling water. Steep 20 minutes, filter, and take small sips during the day. Do not drive or operate machinery. This is very effective for insomnia.

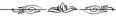

40. Mix one tablespoon each chamomile flowers and European buckthorn bark (*Rhamnus frangula*). To one tablespoon of the mixture, add one cup boiling water. Steep 15 minutes and drink one to two tablespoons before bedtime.

41. Add one tablespoon dill seeds to one cup boiling water. Steep for two hours. Filter and drink ½ cup three times a day 30 minutes before a meal for insomnia accompanied by stomach convulsions or colic.

 42. Put one tablespoon of crushed valerian root in a large glass jar. Add 2½ cups boiling water and steep for two hours. Then filter and drink ½ cup in the morning 30 minutes before a meal. Drink the evening dose with the addition of one teaspoon of honey before bedtime. This is particularly helpful in treating migraine, insomnia, neurosis, irregular heartbeat, and meno-pausal symptoms such as hot flashes.

43. Mix two tablespoons fennel seeds, three tablespoons pep-permint, four tablespoons valerian root, one tablespoon chamomile flowers, and one tablespoon lily of the valley/May lily (*Convallaria majalis*) flowers *or leaves*. Steep one teaspoon of the mixture in one cup cooled boiled water for three hours. Boil again for three minutes, filter, and cool. Drink several times a day in equal portions. It is an excellent natural medicine for insomnia and irregular heartbeat.

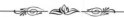

Caution:

Use a heart tonic and diuretic lily of the valley only under the guidance of a qualified practitioner.

44. Mix together one tablespoon wild marjoram, one tablespoon pepper-mint, one teaspoon valerian root, one teaspoon hops, and one tea-spoon rue herb (*Ruta graveolens*). To one tablespoon of the mixture, add one cup spring water. Steep 40 minutes in a warm place. Then filter and drink one tablespoon three times a day 30 minutes before a meal.

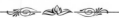

Caution:

Avoid using rue during pregnancy. It is a good circulatory tonic and antispasmodic, but it promotes menstrual flow and lowers blood pressure.

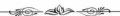

 45. Mix three tablespoons each peppermint, valerian root, bogbean dried leaves *(Menyanthes trifoliata)*. Put one tablespoon of the herbal mixture in a glass jar. Add one cup boiling water. Steep for one hour, filter, and drink one cup three times a day. This drink acts as a sedative and healing medicine for nervous disorders.

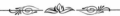

Soak your way to relaxation

 46. A valerian bath: Add eight ounces cut and chopped valerian root to about 24 ounces boiling water. Boil 10 minutes, filter, and pour into the tub. This medicinal bath will soothe your nervous system, decrease excitement in the spinal cord, lower blood pressure, and decrease and regulate the pulse.

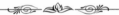

 47. A pine bath: You will need pine needles, twigs, and cones.

    ✒ Full bath = three pounds to five cups water

    ✒ Half-bath = two pounds to four cups water

    ✒ Sit or foot bath = ½ pound to two cups water

In a glass or enamel pot combine pine needles, twigs, cones, and water. Boil 30 minutes, then cover with a lid and steep for two to three hours. Pour into a warm bath. Pine extract should have a rich brown color. This is a very effective remedy for nervous disorders, sleeplessness, and inflammation of the larynx, asthma, pneumonia, and cardiovascular problems.

48. Bathe with the flower from the island of stars. Do you remember the story of chamomile from the previous chapter? That wonderful herb comes to the rescue again! You will need chamomile flowers—fresh or dried.

    ✒ Full bath = one pound to four cups water

    ✒ Half-bath = eight ounces to three cups water

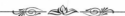

✐ Sit bath = five ounces to two cups water

✐ Foot bath = 4½ ounces to one cup water

Boil the herb in a covered enamel pot with cold water for 10 minutes. Strain and add to bath. A bath of chamomile will alleviate nervousness and emotional stress. The essential oil of chamomile is also used to treat skin inflammation, wounds, and abscesses.

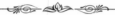

49. A lavender bath: For 10 minutes boil one pound lavender dried flowers in a covered pot with 2½ quarts water. Steep 30 minutes. Add to tub for a healing bath. You'll delight in the fragrance of this healing herb and may experience slight irritation of the skin. There is no cause for worry, however, because the herb is merely increasing activity in the blood vessels. Because of this, it is used to treat cardiac and nervous disorders.

The pharmaceutical industry has addressed the issue of insomnia by providing us with myriad chemical medicines which promise to ensure sleep. Consult your doctor before using them and don't use them for more than two to three weeks in succession. Long-term use of these over-the-counter sleep aids may disrupt your normal sleep pattern and cause nightmares, memory loss, or sexual dysfunction.

All soporific drugs (sedatives) don't depress the functions of the central nervous system. In small doses they act as soporific medicine. In large doses they become narcotics, literally sleep inducers.

When you try self-treatment, you can consider yourself to be your own best friend. Try using natural remedies—innocuous medicines—and have a healthy sleep like a child.

At the beginning of this chapter is an ancient Russian remedy containing hops. People's wisdom is even more extensive than we could ever assume. For instance:

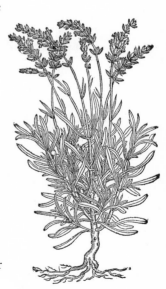

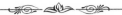

 50. Combine two teaspoons of hops flowers in a glass jar with eight ounces boiling water. Cover with a lid and steep four hours. Filter and drink one cup before bed.

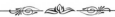

 51. Combine one teaspoon minced hops flowers with four ounces vodka or white grape juice in a covered jar. Steep it in a dark place for two weeks. Filter and take five drops in a tablespoon of boiled water, twice before eating and once before bed.

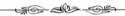

 52. Dill tincture. Combine two ounces dill seeds and one pint Port wine in an enamel pot. Simmer 15-20 minutes. Steep one hour, filter, and drink ¼ cup before bed.

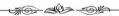

 53. "Southern Night" balm. Mix one teaspoon lemon balm, dried or fresh leaves (Melissa officinalis), two teaspoons dried rose hips berries (Rosa canina), two teaspoons eucalyptus leaves, two twigs juniper (minced), three teaspoons sage, and three teaspoons thyme. Combine minced herbs in a thermos with one quart boiling water and steep for six hours. Filter. Pour balm into an atomizer. Mist bedroom with the balm. The effect of this natural medicine will be enhanced if combined with an evening walk before bedtime and a relaxing self-massage.

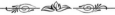

Calming tea blends

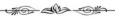

 54. Mix one tablespoon valerian root, two tablespoons mint leaves, one tablespoon hops flowers, and two tablespoons yarrow. Combine one tablespoon of this herbal mixture in a porcelain bowl with two cups boiling water. Cover and steep 30 minutes. Filter, add one tablespoon honey, and drink four ounces once in the morning and once before bed. This is especially effective in the treatment of nervous excitement or irritability.

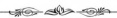

The following four recipes are prepared by steeping the specified amount of herb in one quart boiled water for 10 minutes in a covered pot. Filter and enjoy!

 55. Try two tablespoons of one of the following: peppermint leaves, fennel seeds, valerian root, chamomile flowers, or caraway seeds. Drink one to two cups in the morning and before bed.

 56. Combine three tablespoons chamomile flowers, five tablespoons caraway seeds, and two tablespoons valerian root. Drink one to two cups in the morning and before bed.

 57. Steep together the following: three tablespoons peppermint leaves, three tablespoons motherwort leaves, two tablespoons valerian root, and two tablespoons hops flowers. Drink four ounces three times daily.

 58. Mix two tablespoons horsetail (dried aerial parts), three tablespoons knotgrass/bird's buckwheat herb, and five tablespoons hawthorn flowering tops. Sip two ounces of the tea twice a day.

Vitamin-rich teas

Method of preparation: Combine in a pot two tablespoons of the mixed herbs with two cups boiling water. Steep 10 minutes. Filter. Drink one to two cups hot herbal tea daily.

 59. 4½ tablespoons rose hips
four tablespoons nettle
1½ tablespoons cranberries

 60. Three tablespoons rose hips
One tablespoon black currant
Three tablespoons nettle
Three tablespoons minced carrot

After you've successfully treated yourself with a healing remedy and you are feeling better, try these cheerful libations:

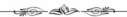

 61. Sunny Berry Punch. Grate peel of one lemon. Whip with 12–14 ounces honey and one quart white wine. Boil 10 minutes. Add 3 ounces cognac or rum. Enjoy a glass of hot punch.

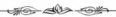

 62. Milk Punch. Grate peel of one lemon and blend with one pound honey. Add one quart white Chardonnay wine and one pint fresh skim milk. Whip well to thicken. Boil five to seven minutes with two ounces crushed almonds and a dash of vanilla. Filter and fill glass half full. Top with whipped cream. Your punch is ready to cheer you up.

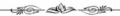

 63. Cold Punch. Mix 24 ounces of honey with grated dried peel of one lemon. Add 1½ quarts white Chardonnay wine, juice of one lemon, one ounce cognac, a dash of vanilla, and one cup cold boiled water. Mix well, filter, and pour into bottles. This punch will keep several days in your refrigerator. From time to time, use it as a mood enhancer and sleep inducer.

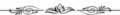

The above concoctions are small "miracles" in our lives, made from the properties of blessed herbs and plants.

In the Russian folk tale, "The Tale of the Firebird, Tsarevich Ivan and the Gray Wolf," a larger miracle takes place. Let me tell you how a mysterious firebird easily induced sound sleep into those she met (much better than any doctor could do—and she didn't resort to prescribing fast-acting sleeping pills).

*O*nce upon a time in a far-off land lived a Russian tsar in a magnificent palace on the side of a mountain. His palace garden was so beautiful, none could find a better one anywhere in the world. It was home to thousands of aromatic flowers, gigantic trees, and lush plants. Among the most notable trees was an unusually tall apple tree, which bestowed upon the tsar a daily harvest of magnificent golden fruit. This tree was his favorite and ranked among his beloved treasures.

As time passed, the tsar noticed that many of his apples began disappearing overnight. His servants told of a large and beautiful firebird that plucked the apples from the tree branches every evening as the royal court slumbered. The tsar called his three sons, Tsarevich Dimitri, Tsarevich Vasily, and Tsarevich Ivan, and told them that the firebird had been stealing his golden apples and made a bargain with them. "If one of you will capture the firebird alive, I'll give you half of my kingdom while I live and the rest of it upon my death."

His three sons listened to him with great respect and vowed that one of them would indeed capture the bird and place it alive at the feet of their father. The oldest son, Tsarevich Dimitri, went into the garden the first night to watch for the firebird. He sat under the wide wreath of golden apples that crowned the apple tree, and as the night drew on, he became drowsy and fell into a deep sleep. While he slept peacefully, the firebird flew into the garden, picked as many apples as she wished, and flew away.

In the morning the tsar asked Dimitri if he had seen the firebird. Dimitri answered that she never came into the garden that night. The second night Tsarevich Vasily kept watch in the garden. He sat under the apple tree as his brother had, and after several hours of waiting in darkness and silence, he too fell asleep. The next morning Vasily told the tsar that the firebird had not visited the garden.

The third night, the youngest tsar's son, Tsarevich Ivan, assumed his post in the garden to watch for the firebird. He sat under the apple tree as his older brothers had done the previous two nights. For the first several hours, nothing happened. All was quiet until suddenly the garden was illuminated by a brilliant golden light.

The firebird soared into the garden, her eyes sparkling like two faceted crystals, her wings streaming golden flames. She lit on a branch of the apple tree and began to tug at and pluck the juicy apples. Tsarevich

Ivan stole up quietly and tried to catch her, but the firebird was strong and he wasn't able to hold on to her, even as he clasped her magnificent tail in both of his hands. The firebird tore herself from his grasp, leaving behind only one incredibly beautiful feather in his hands.

In the morning Ivan met with his father and gave him the firebird's feather. The tsar was pleased that finally one of his three sons had succeeded if not in catching the firebird, at least in getting one of her feathers. He brought this feather into his royal chamber and instantly the entire palace glowed as though lighted by thousands of radiant candles.

From that time on, the firebird never again returned to the garden, but the tsar had become obsessed by his desire to have her in his palace.

To make a long story short, I can tell you briefly that the tsar's three sons had many adventures in their quest for the firebird. Tsarevich Ivan met a gray wolf which served him as a mighty stead and he fell madly in love with a beautiful princess named Elena. He eventually captured the firebird, put her in a golden cage, and set off with Princess Elena to his father's palace. But the way to his homeland was a long journey, and the two lovers with the firebird, stopped to rest near the forest and fell asleep. As they slept, Ivan's jealous brothers killed him, stole the firebird and his magic horse with the golden mane, kidnapped his beautiful bride, and arrived at the tsar's palace as great heroes. But this would not be a fairy tale if it didn't have a happy ending.

So here's what happened next. Tsarevich Ivan lay dead for 30 days until his friend, the gray wolf, found him and sprinkled his body with the water of life. Tsarevich Ivan stood up in a twinkle of an eye.

"I have slept for a long time," he said.

"Yes," answered the wolf, "you would have slept forever if I had not brought you back to life."

Then he told him how his brothers had slain him. In a fairy tale, truth and justice always prevail, so Ivan's brothers could not believe their eyes when they saw Tsarevich Ivan alive. They lost their peace of mind and became sick with insomnia. They never could fall asleep at night anymore.

Meanwhile Tsarevich Ivan was blessed with a sound and healthy sleep forevermore. He married the beautiful Elena … and, of course, they lived happily ever after.

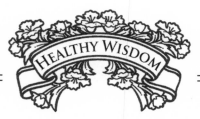

If you can't sleep, then get up and do something instead of lying there and worrying. It's the worry that gets you, not the loss of sleep.

—Dale Carnegie (1855–1955), How to Win Friends and Influence People

Health is the first muse, and sleep is the condition to produce it.

—Ralph Waldo Emerson (1803–1882), American poet and essayist

A well-spent day brings happy sleep.

—Leonardo Da Vinci (1452–1519), Florentine artist and scientist

Sleep . . . peace of the soul, who puts test care to flight.

—Ovid (43 B.C.–A.D. 18), Latin poet

There is a fullness of all things, even of sleep and of love.

—Homer (700 B.C.), Greek poet, author of The Iliad and The Odyssey

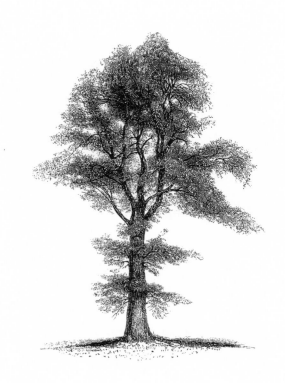

Chapter 9

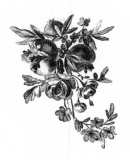

When Your Head Is Swimming

Nature is not a competition. It doesn't really matter, when you go out,
if you don't identify anything. What matters is the feeling heart.

—*Richard Adams (b.1920), British writer*

FACTS

How large is the problem of fatigue? According to a recent Department of Health and Human Services report entitled "Reasons for Visiting Physicians," a staggering 14 million Americans go to the doctor complaining of exhaustion. Add to that uncounted millions who seek medical advice for other reasons but also mention significant exhaustion. There are millions more who seek help but are nonetheless tired all the time. It becomes clear that fatigue is one of the major health problems in America. Many years ago in Alameda County, California, only 6 percent of the adult population qualified as energetic and healthy.[30]

"Generally speaking, the dictionary defines *fatigue* with equally incomplete substitutes such as tiredness, lassitude, exhaustion, ennui, burnout, and/or boredom. Some few larger lexicons go beyond this synonym chanting. When they do, fatigue and energy are somehow related. As energy goes down, fatigue goes up! According to the International Classification of Diseases, fatigue is now recognized as a sovereign syndrome with its own distinctive designation (Chronic Fatigue Syndrome), its abbreviation (CFS), and its own number (780.7)."[31]

hen we are overtired, we may experience headaches and sleeplessness, but also giddiness, or so-called swimming head or dizziness. Dizziness is usually caused by an irregular distribution of blood to different parts of the brain. Dizziness may be associated with a variety of ailments including stress, high blood pressure, constipation, and high acidity in the stomach. It may be accompanied by nausea. If so, it's important to cleanse the stomach.

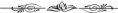

1. A very good way to cleanse the stomach is with a chamomile enema. See page 70, R59., for instructions. Allow the enema to aid in elimination of toxins and then lie down on a bed in a darkened room and close your eyes. Place an ice bag on your forehead and relax.

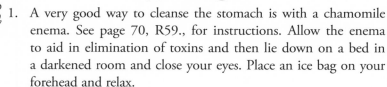

2. If dizziness is a result of overwork, try the following mix: 1½ tablespoons each of hawthorn berries and hawthorn flowers, and three cups boiling water. Steep for two hours in a warm place. Filter. Drink three times daily 30 minutes before any meal or one hour after eating or whenever you feel dizzy.

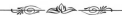

3. Mix one tablespoon hawthorn berries and one cup boiling water. Steep two hours in a warm spot, preferably a preheated warm oven. Filter and take one to two tablespoons three to four times daily prior to eating.

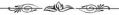

4. Drink one cup of potato juice to neutralize acidity in the stomach.

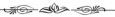

5. Make mint drops. This medicine will have the same effect as potato juice, but in addition it will disinfect and warm the internal organs. It will help eliminate heartburn and relieve stomach gas. Mince one tablespoon of mint leaves. Combine in a glass jar with ½ cup 90 percent alcohol (vodka). Cover and steep overnight, shaking it periodically. Filter and add one tablespoon mint oil. Take five drops of mint tincture twice daily.

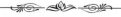

6. Take three to five drops of mint tincture (see #5) on a sugar cube or dissolve the mint tincture in one tablespoon boiled water. I remember that we always had two vital vials in our domestic pharmacy, one prepared by Grandma or Mama, both of whom preferred to make the remedies themselves rather than buy them in a drugstore. Mint drops were always "friendly" natural medicines and good aids in healing the diseases I mentioned above.

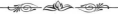

 7. Try to clean the blood and improve your digestion by paying close attention to the food you eat. Learn to balance a healthy diet of fish, eggs, cheese, and vegetables, especially radishes, cucumbers, green peas, and walnuts, which contain phosphorus. Phosphorus is a main component of cerebral substance and its quantity decreases with strenuous brain work. We have to replenish our body with this mineral to safeguard against Alzheimer's disease and strokes.

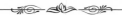

If you are bothered by excess stomach acidity, try the following people's medicines. They are simple but reliable and effective natural methods.

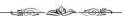

 8. Make *Aurica* Drink to balance stomach acids. Mix two tablespoons minced calendula (pot marigold) flowers and two tablespoons minced blackberry leaves. Add one quart boiling water and let steep in preheated but cooling oven overnight. Filter in the morning. Drink three cups daily. This simple people's remedy is a favorite of mine and very effective. Aurica Drink is also a tonic for energy in recovery from illness.

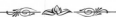

 9. Mix one tablespoon sage, one tablespoon peppermint, and ½ teaspoon cinnamon. Combine all herbs in a china bowl with 4½ cups boiling water. Steep for 20 minutes. Drink ½ cup of this medicinal drink daily for two weeks to treat stomach acidity. Repeat the same course after six months.

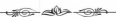

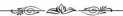

10. Take systematically 600 mg to 1,200 mg. calcium daily. Calcium is a necessary addition to the diet not only for healthy bones but also to ensure proper functioning of the liver, pancreas, tonsils, and endocrine and other glands supplying hormones to the blood, tissues, and cells.

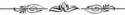

11. Make a habit of drinking chamomile or peppermint tea on an empty stomach in the mornings. Combine one teaspoon of the herbs in #8 or #9 in a glass jar with one cup boiling water and steep for 15 minutes. Drink once in the morning.

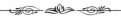

When I was a little girl, Mama would prepare for me before bed a glass of fresh warm milk from our cow. To the milk she would add a teaspoon of honey—nothing more. This simple remedy gave me a sound sleep filled with colorful dreams. I called them "sleepy movies" and they were full of happy events and noble actions.

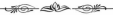

12. Drink a glass of fresh warm milk with one teaspoon of honey before you go to bed and you'll have a sound sleep.

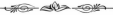

However, if you want to have energy, do what Hippocrates widely advised more than 2,400 years ago: "Let food be thy medicine." His food therapy principle is incorporated into plant therapy. Through the modern conception and use of this idea, body sicknesses have been miraculously corrected.

Dr. Ann Wigmore, founder of the Hippocrates Health Institute, now worldwide in scope, wrote in her book, *Be Your Own Doctor (Let Living Food Be Your Medicine)*: "Through long and careful observation of myself and others, I found that when we give our bodies the rich nourishment they need from living foods, and, when we work in close harmony with Nature's laws, Nature's boundless healing power will always be there to assist us."

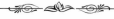

13. Nourish yourself and make buckwheat kasha with sour cream, plain yogurt, or warm milk in the morning, at lunch, or at

dinner, but no later than 6:00 P. M. It'll give you a light living food filled with vitamins.

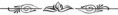

Although not very popular in the United States, buckwheat has been used as a food by Europeans for centuries. It is also grown in northern America but has not yet gained much recognition and popularity among American consumers. Buckwheat becomes a superior salad lettuce when it is grown for seven days.

The Russian word for buckwheat is *grechikha*. Let's assume that the ancient Slavs adopted buckwheat from Greeks who lived since olden times on the shores of the Black Sea. This plant was widely cultivated in Russia and other European countries from the fifteenth century, but in the United States it is used primarily as food for cattle and a cereal grain. Buckwheat's nutritional value is unprecedented. It is rich in iron, calcium, phosphorous, copper, boron, iodine, and other minerals.

The well-respected pharmaceutical industry produces rutin, using buckwheat leaves and flowers. Rutin is the same preparation as vitamin P, which is an irreplaceable treatment for those affected by radiation and sclerosis, hypertension, stoke, bleeding, rheumatism, nephritis, glaucoma, measles, and nervous disorders. As you see, it boasts a wide spectrum of healing properties.

I have observed for many years that in the United States elderly people are familiar with this plant and its benefits. My guess is they were taught about it by their European ancestors. But few young people have been introduced to buckwheat meals by their mothers or grandmothers.

I purchase buckwheat in a local health-food market and often prepare kasha with sour cream, milk, or yogurt for my family as a nutritious breakfast. They love it.

Buckwheat is one of the most important plants for maintaining good health. It is a source of high energy and amazing health. And more good news is that it is low in calories and satisfies the appetite.

Buckwheat whole grains (groats) are used to make porridge or *kasha*, as it is called in Russia. In common parlance it is called *grechka*. But I want to warn you that not everybody will like the taste of this meal. It is meatless and not everyone will consider it a "real" food. Even children can turn up their noses at this meal, and they will do it again and again until they acquire a taste for it and begin to understand its superior nutritional value.

Kasha is "the original mother of bread" and it has been known and used widely throughout the world for more than a thousand years. Try it and make a delightful breakfast, lunch, or dinner. You will be giving your body the gift of rich nourishment and the key to energy, health, and longevity.

Here are eight delicious recipes:

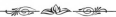

 14. Buckwheat friable kasha. Lightly roast one cup of whole grain buckwheat in a pan in the oven for about three minutes. Put buckwheat into two cups of boiling water. Add a pinch of salt. Return to a boil, then reduce heat and cook until the water is gone and the buckwheat is soft and ready to eat, approximately 20 minutes. Mix in two teaspoons of butter or olive oil and cover. Serve kasha with sour cream, salsa, or milk. If you decide to use only milk, add a teaspoon of honey. It makes a healthy breakfast, which can be a nutritious part of your diet. You can add friable buckwheat kasha as an easy-to-make, light nutritional side dish, complimenting meat, fish, or chicken for lunch or dinner.

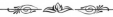

 15. "Downy" kasha for children. Rinse one cup buckwheat whole grains in a sieve. Mix in a bowl with one egg and place the mixture on the griddle or dry it in an oven on a pan about three minutes at 375°. Boil two cups milk and add one tablespoon of butter, a pinch of salt, and the dried buckwheat. Reduce heat and continue to cook. Kasha will be ready to eat in 15-20 minutes. Serve it with a sweet milk sauce over it: Dissolve one teaspoon starch in one tablespoon of cold milk or water. Add one cup milk and bring to a boil. Add one teaspoon sugar or honey and bring again to a boil for two to three minutes. Add 1/4 teaspoon vanilla or vanilla sugar. The sweet milk sauce will bring a tender taste to a "downy" kasha. I can assure you the children will love it.

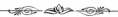

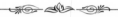

16. Buckwheat kasha with cheese. Wash and pass ½ cup buckwheat whole grains through a sieve. Pour one cup water into a pot. Add a pinch of salt and bring to a boil. Then add buckwheat to the boiling water and cook until thickened, approximately 20 minutes. Reduce heat. Add one teaspoon of butter when kasha is almost ready. Mix well and cover. Place the pot with buckwheat in a bigger pan with hot water and continue to cook in this water bath for 15 minutes more. Loosen kasha with a fork and mound it on a plate. Pour on melted butter. Strew three to four ounces of friable Farmers cheese or any other cheese like an authentic Greek feta cheese, Mozzarella, or baby cheese on top. Sprinkle with chopped dill or parsley and garnish with ¼ sliced tomato.

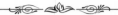

17. Sailor's kasha. Cook a friable buckwheat kasha (as in #14), using two cups buckwheat whole grains and four cups water. Cut one pound veal in small pieces, wash it well, then grind it. Fry two to three shredded onions in a frying pan with olive oil. Boil two eggs. Let them cool, then shred them. Mix ground veal, fried onions, a dash of black pepper, and shredded eggs to the kasha. Then oil a three-quart pan and place prepared mixture inside. Let it stew in a 350° oven until ready, about 25 minutes. Sailor's kasha is one of the best nutritious meals, served hot for lunch or dinner.

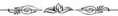

18. "Shrimp" kasha. Cook friable kasha (as in #14), using two cups buckwheat whole grains and four cups water. Add two tablespoons butter, pinch of salt, two teaspoons minced garlic, one tablespoon dill or parsley, and four ounces cooked popcorn shrimp. This makes a healthy dinner for four to six people.

19. Kasha Soufflé. Wash two cups buckwheat grains and place into a pot with four cups boiling water. Cook until softened, approximately 15-20 minutes. Then rub kasha through a sieve. Add one teaspoon honey or sugar, a pinch of salt, and ½ cup milk. Cook an additional two to three minutes, mixing constantly. Remove from stove and add ½ teaspoon butter, mixing well. It is excellent as a breakfast, lunch, or light dinner.

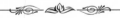

Buckwheat has been so well respected in Europe for centuries that Hans Christian Andersen also became interested in this plant. Writing a story about buckwheat, he confessed, "This is the story told me by the sparrows one evening when I begged them to relate some tale to me."

"Very often after a violent thunderstorm, a field of buckwheat appears blackened and singed, as if a flame of fire passed over it. The country people say that this appearance is caused by lightning; but I will tell you what the sparrow says, and the sparrow heard it from an old willow-tree which grew near a field of buckwheat, and is there still. It is a large venerable tree, though a little crippled by age. The trunk has been split, and out of the crevice grass and brambles grow. The tree bends forward slightly, and the branches hang quite down to the ground just like green hair. Corn grows in the surrounding fields, not only rye and barley, but oats—pretty oats that, when ripe, look like a number of little golden canary birds, sitting on a bough. The corn has a smiling look and the heaviest and richest ears bend their heads low as if in pious humility. Once there was also a field of buckwheat, and this field was exactly opposite the old willow-tree. The buckwheat did not bend like the other grain, but erected its head proudly and stiffly on the stem.

"'I am as valuable as any other corn,' said he, 'and I am much handsomer; my flowers are as beautiful as the bloom of the apple blossom, and it is a pleasure to look at us. Do you know of anything prettier than we are, you old willow-tree?'

And the willow-tree nodded his head, as if he would say, 'Indeed I do.'

But the buckwheat spread itself out with pride, and said, 'Stupid tree; he is so old that grass grows out of his body.'"

There arose a very terrible storm. All the field flowers folded their leaves together, or bowed their little heads, while the storm passed over them, but the buckwheat stood erect in its pride. 'Bend your head as we do,' said the flowers.

"'I have no occasion to do so,' replied the buckwheat.

"'Bend your head as we do,' cried the ears of corn. 'The angel of the storm is coming; his wings spread from the sky above the earth beneath. He will stroke you down before you can cry for mercy.'

"'But I will not bend my head,' said the buckwheat.

"'Close your flowers and bend your leaves,' said the old willow-tree. 'Do not look at the lightning when the cloud bursts; even men cannot do that. In a flash of lightning heaven opens, and we can look in; but the sight will strike even human beings blind. What then must happen to us, who only grow out of the earth, and are so inferior to them, if we venture to do so?'

"'Inferior, indeed!' said the buckwheat. 'Now I intend to have a peep into heaven.' Proudly and boldly he looked up, while the lightning flashed across the sky as if the whole world were in flames.

"When the dreadful storm passed, the flowers and the corn raised their drooping heads in the pure still air, refreshed by the rain, but the buckwheat lay like a weed in the field, burnt to blackness by the lightning. The branches of the old willow-tree rustled in the wind, and large water-drops fell from his green leaves as if the old willow were weeping. Then the sparrows asked why he was weeping, when all around him seemed so cheerful. 'See,' they said, 'how the sun shines, and the clouds float in the blue sky. Do you not smell the sweet perfume from flower or bush? Wherefore do you weep, old willow-tree?'

"Then the willow tree told them of the haughty pride of the buckwheat, and of the punishment which followed in consequence."

So you see, the buckwheat can be unreasonable sometimes, but it always brings people its best nutritious values. And you can count on him without reservation, he will not disappoint you.

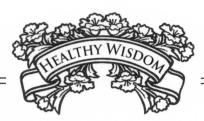

Before you trust a man, eat a peck of salt with him.

—Russian proverb

One should eat to live—not live to eat.

—Benjamin Franklin (1706-1790), American statesman, printer, and inventor

Unquiet meals make ill digestion.

—Shakespeare, The Comedy of Errors

The belly will not listen to advice.

—Seneca, Epistulae ad Lucilium

Nothing in excess. Nihil nimis.

—Latin saying

Chapter 10

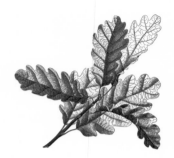

Don't Be Afraid of Good Stress

It is not enough only to wish; you must also act.

—*Johann Wolfgang von Goethe (1749-1832), German poet and novelist*

FACTS:

Stress is both additive and cumulative in its negative effects on individuals, organizations, and societies. Workplace stress continues to grow. In the United States experts at the Centers of Disease Control and the National Institute for Occupational Safety and Healthcare are dedicated to studying stress. They found that $300 billion, or $7,500 per employee, is spent annually in the United States on stress-related compensation claims, reduced productivity, absenteeism, health insurance costs, direct medical expenses (nearly 50 percent or higher for workers who report stress), and employee turnover.

Stress affects physical and mental health, and is linked to a decreased willingness to take on new and creative endeavors, and job burnout, which is experienced by 25–40 percent of U. S. workers. More than ever before, employee stress is being recognized as a major drain on corporate productivity and competitiveness.

Statistics from a recent global stress research study show that increased stress is felt worldwide, and stress affects women differently than men. Women who work full-time and have children under age 13 report the greatest stress. Nearly one in four mothers who work full-time and have children under age 13 feel stress. Globally 23 percent of women executives and professionals say they feel "super-stressed."[32]

On spring break from Moscow State University I came home exhausted. I had undergone a grueling winter session of many exams, which would determine my eligibility to remain in classes for the second half of the school year.

When I arrived at the airport, Mama took a look at me and shook her head in disapproval. I couldn't blame her. I felt as if all my energy was spent, and as I listened to my body, it sometimes seemed to me that my blood had difficulty circulating through my veins and blood vessels.

"Oh, oh!" I thought while grinning at Mama. "Our family doctor (Mama) has found herself a new patient." Mama always worried about me and she was always overprotective.

I knew intuitively that I was due for a course of Mama's vitamin therapy. She frowned at me and said, "Are you running out of energy? I can tell without testing that your hemoglobin level is very low. You need a special course of vitamins."

"Didn't I read her thoughts?" I asked myself.

Milk with rose hips jam or rose hips preserves was an "urgent remedy" in Mama's list of natural treatments. And the manufacturer of those tasty natural remedies was Grandma. Each year Grandma made delicious preserves, jams, and other natural delights from rose hips as well as grapes, plums, strawberries, raspberries, black and red currants, cranberries, cherries, gooseberries, peaches, small "paradise apples," pears, apricots, green nuts, oranges, and quinces.

She cooked exotic preserves from green tomatoes, green beans, watermelon rind, and pumpkin cooked in a grape mousse. My favorite, and the most prescribed by Mama, was rose hips and black currant preserves.

Black currants are an important ingredient in vitamin therapy. We called these berries *Ribes* from the Latin, *Ribes Nigrum* or *Chernaya Smorodina*. Grandma grew this shrub in her garden. A medium-sized shrub with yellow-brown shoots, five-lobed leaves, and green-white flowers, this bush bore many berry clusters annually. This berry is less common in the United States because it can host pine blister rust (*Cronartium Ribicola*), which can devastate forests. It is more readily available now because of recent commercial breeding.

Grandma used large, plump berries in her delicious black currant preserves. She combined 32 ounces of honey or two pounds of sugar, 16 ounces of water, and two pounds of black currants. Then she cooked the mixture until it thickened, periodically removing the froth that formed during cooking. It was a tasty preserve that complemented our black or green teas.

I always tasted these preserves as soon as she finished preparing them. Just imagine tasting a spoonful of this 100-percent natural, indigo mixture thick with tiny grains of rubbed berries and following it with a sip of hot, aromatic Ceylon tea. It is so delicious!

In shady places throughout Grandma's garden stood thorny shrubs of rose hips. She plucked fragrant petals from the flowers and boiled them in water for two to three minutes. Then she added lemon juice, covered the mixture with a lid, and steeped it for 15–20 minutes. Then she poured the pink rose juice into a pot with the preserves along with sugar or honey to make syrup.

If you'd like to try this recipe, prepare 10 ounces rose hips petals, two pounds sugar or 24 ounces honey, two tablespoons lemon juice, and eight ounces water.

Grandma also made a tasty jam from the raw pulp of rose hips, ground with honey or sugar.

She would cook rose hips berries as a special medicinal preserve, knowing that rose hips contain almost 40 percent of vitamin C, and are, therefore, a valuable vitamin product.

Concoctions, preserves, and jams from wild roses or rose hips (*shipovnik*) berries that Grandma had dried herself were also mainstays in our home. Over a campfire in our backyard, she would boil four pounds of fresh berries in their own juice for 10 minutes. She then mashed the berry mixture and cooked it in a water bath until it thickened. Her water-bath method was to sink the small pan containing rose hips pulp into a large pan of boiling water.

In our kitchen we always had a glass pitcher filled with rose hips or "Dog Rose" concoction (*otvar*). You can make it yourself by following these directions:

Boil one tablespoon of fresh rose hips (also called wild roses) in about eight ounces of water for seven or eight minutes. Allow to steep for two hours. Or combine a half-ounce of *dried* rose hips berries with eight ounces of water. Boil seven or eight minutes and allow to steep for 10 hours. Then drink four to eight ounces of this vitamin tea daily.

Mama prescribed for me a 24-hour healing session of rose hips preserves and black currant preserves, fruit compotes and *kissels,* which is a kind of starchy jelly. I took teaspoon after teaspoon of Grandma's thick burgundy rose hips preserves. And, with every sip of tea and every spoonful of cold black currant preserves, energy poured through my body and I actually felt my blood begin to circulate with intensity through my veins.

I felt much better later as I stood in our kitchen watching the sunlight peep into the window while several branches of a rose bush, encouraged by a gentle breeze, tapped gently on the windowpanes. Each year the roses took full advantage of the sun and blossomed again and again. The sunbeams traveled like a beacon through the kitchen window, rode over the ceiling, and then stopped, blinding me.

A bouquet of velvety scarlet and white roses followed the sunbeams and appeared outside the kitchen window. Someone had come to visit. I looked out and saw that my neighbor and long-time friend, Sasha, had come to say hello. He was always happy to see me when I came home for vacation. I suspected that Grandma had been giving him reports on when I'd return home and how long I would stay. She admired his decency, kindness, and his good looks.

"Hi, Sasha. How have you survived here without me?" I asked him alluringly as always whenever I returned home.

And, in turn, he teased me as usual. "Obviously I am doing badly without you!"

"How did you know I was here?" I asked coyly, guessing that he would say that Grandma had told him.

From the doorstep he answered me with a smile, "Do you know that a wireless telegraph company just opened its first office in our town? It helps guys like me find hidden and unsupportive friends."

Sasha, still smiling, shook a red and white bouquet of fragrant roses at me. He used his charm and gestured to me to come outside to talk for a minute. I wrote him a note that I pressed against the windowpane: "Later. I don't know when." I didn't await his reply, but returned to my room to read a book. I read for a short while and then dropped off to sleep. I don't know how many hours passed, but when I woke up, I saw on the floor near my bed the same bouquet of roses. I took the bouquet in my hands and breathed in its soft, sweet fragrance. A small note written in old script was tucked inside: "Here are my flowers and here is my heart, which beats only for you."

That was a day filled with both *dis*tress and "good" stress. Let's take a look at how Mama differentiated between the two types of stress.

Making stress work for you

We have seen that stress is the impetus behind many neuroses and cardiovascular problems. Mama would have added, "Don't be afraid of stress. Make it work for you, not against you."

How can we manage tension in our everyday lives when it results from unhappiness with our jobs or the relationships we have with our children, our friends, or spouse?

Take a look at the way stress influences yourself and others. Heightened tension is common among most of us. It seems that many people do everything with a great amount of unnecessary effort. Even the simple act of listening to others is difficult for most people and often met with anxiousness or uneasiness—the result of too much unmanaged stress, no doubt.

Most people do not know how to control stress. Do you know how to recognize stress and how to control it?

Typical symptoms of stress are chronic headaches, high blood pressure, tightness in the chest, sleeplessness, or restless sleep.

Mama always advised her patients, "Don't be afraid of stress. Learn how to recognize it." Mama knew that we experience stress on a physical level as well as on mental and psychological levels. She also taught us to differentiate between *healthy* stress and *dis*tress.

Happiness and even the *anticipation* of a happy event such as the birth of a baby are stresses, but certainly they are positive stresses. This kind of stress doesn't promote illness. On the contrary, it brings about and maintains positive emotional and physical strength. Mama called this stress "a good exercise for heart and soul."

Distress is different. Distress is experienced in emotional, epigastria, fetal, mental, and respiratory forms. All too often, when people talk about stress, what they are actually referring to is *dis*tress.

Distress is defined by resulting feelings of discontent, dissatisfaction, and irritation. Distress is caused by many things, including arguments between spouses or lovers or between parents and children.

Ups and downs in our lives are normal, frequent occurrences. At times, though, it can feel as though life demands too much and that we do not have any time to relax and to ease or even eliminate the tension and stress we have stored throughout the week.

As we scurry around tending to our often overwhelming responsibilities, it seems that we have run out of time to tend to ourselves. The *stress* we were feeling has become *distress*.

Is there a method to combat the stress before it becomes distress? Yes! Learn to recognize stress and devise your own personal methods to gain control over it. It does not have to be difficult to manage stress before it manages you. It simply takes a little planning.

Five simple guidelines will help you to recover from distress and rebalance your internal, psychological health. Interpret these concepts in your personal way, add new ones of your own, and minimize the harmful effects of stress on your well-being.

A. Practice proper nutrition

Scientists and physicians confirm that eating a balanced diet, low in fat and rich in vitamins and nutrients, is a powerful defense against the toll that stress can take on us.

Magnesium is an important mineral that relieves muscle cramping and strengthens blood vessels and the heart. Dizziness, high blood pressure, trembling, and itching of the fingers can be an indication of a magnesium deficiency in the body. To ensure that your body has sufficient magnesium, try Mama's simple remedies:

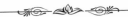

 1.   Drink a good quality mineral water.

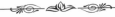 2.   Eat plenty of fresh fruits and vegetables.

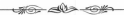

3. Take a daily dose of magnesium by eating a mixture of two to three freshly grated carrots with a minced onion in a little light olive oil.

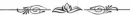

4. At least twice weekly make yourself a glass of fresh carrot juice. It's a strong blood purifier and will help to cleanse the body of physical and psychological impurities.

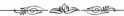

5. Make herbal tea, which Mama would say "relieves the soul of tension." This combination of herbs is to be taken once in the morning and evening. Mix one teaspoon each thyme, sage, and linden. Add one pint of boiling water and steep for five minutes. Filter and add honey to taste. Sip this beverage slowly and enjoy.

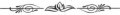

B. Use hydrotherapy to combat distress

Our bathrooms can be a sensual departure from the day-to-day grind—a haven of joy in which we can experience peace and serenity.

6. Take a warm shower or bath with 16 ounces of apple cider vinegar mixed with eight ounces of water (to reduce acidity). Cleansing your skin with this mixture will open pores and draw out toxins. Your skin will feel smoother and you will feel relaxed.

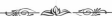

7. For a soothing self-massage, soak a linen towel in hot water, wring it out, and rub your body vigorously with it. Begin on the soles of your feet and direct the motion toward your heart. Afterwards, massage your body with pine extract. You will experience increased blood circulation and your skin will have a rosy glow. As you lie in bed, you will experience a warm sensation over your body.

8. Another great benefit for the body is to massage your skin with a dry-skin brush, which can be purchased at a health-food store. Each morning massage the body in circular motions with the brush or a cotton mitten. Mama said, "It provides the body with

Don't Be Afraid of Good Stress 🥄 191

a fair distribution of blood." What she meant by that statement is that a dry massage promotes proper distribution of blood to our internal organs and thus better blood circulation overall.

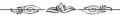

Relax or energize by bathing with aromatherapy

After a busy day, try one of these:

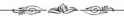

 9. Fill a vase with your favorite beautiful fresh flowers. Turn off the bright electric bulbs and light an aromatic candle instead. Allow it to burn at least 10 minutes before you bathe to ensure that the herbal aroma, which is so beneficial in relaxing the nervous system, fills the room. Add to the bath aromatic mineral salts or an essential oil such as rose, jasmine, or bergamot. Tie up a handful of dried lavender flowers or fresh rose petals in a scrap of lace or gauze and toss into the water. A warm bath of just 15 minutes can be sufficient in relieving distress. After bathing, massage your skin with a cotton towel, and slather on a rich moisturizing cream before retiring.

 10. An herbal bath can relax or rejuvenate. A bath of 20 drops of essential oil of chamomile or calendula, for example, is known to cleanse the skin and calm the nervous system. Or put a twist on a simple chamomile bath by mixing just 10 drops of chamomile with 10 drops of lavender and eight drops of sage and feel the day's troubles float away with the bath water. Only add neat oils to bathwater if they are guaranteed to be non-irritants, such as Roman chamomile and lavender. Otherwise dilute the oil in carrier oil such as apricot kernel or sweet almond. Five drops of jojoba oil can be added for very dry skin. Then swirl the bathwater around and the oils will be dispersed before you step into the bath. These oils added to bathwater are inhaled and partly absorbed by the skin, bringing immediate physical relief.

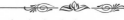

 11. Aromatic essential oils, bath foams, and candles are instrumental in helping to impart a sense of luxury and beauty and induce

a feeling of serenity and comfort. Aromas are generally divided into two categories: those that stimulate and those that relax.

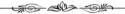

Stimulating aromas include peppermint, anise, eucalyptus, lemon, rosemary, pine, cinnamon, cardamom, camphor, and nutmeg.

Relaxing aromas include bergamot, chamomile, sandalwood, jasmine, cypress, lavender, juniper, rose, lemon balm, orange, and honeysuckle.

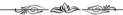

 12. The therapeutic potential of classical music has long been recognized. Lower the volume on the stereo and allow your favorite classical music to waft softly through the air. You might choose Mozart, Strauss, Tchaikovsky, Chopin, or Vivaldi. Listen to gentle, relaxing music. It will calm you down in times of stress and make you feel better about yourself.

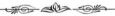

C. Move your body! Exercise!

Walk or jog. Swim or run. Find a sport or activity that moves you—and move! Dance, dance, dance as often as you have a chance! Dance is a pleasant physical exercise which allows us to express our emotions through movement. A popular aphorism in Europe is: Those who dance a lot live a lot. When we feel comfortable in our lives, we win the fight with distress.

When I found out I had been accepted as a new student at Moscow State University, I was overjoyed. But at the same time I had a plaintive feeling that something very close and familiar was missing from my life. Certainly, as a freshman far from home, I missed my family and the whole environment in which I grew up. My head was swimming, and I couldn't have guessed then, but now I know I was suffering from distress.

> *Caution:*
>
> Seek professional advice before using essential oils if you have a long-standing medical condition such as asthma, heart disease, high blood pressure, or diabetes. People who are allergy prone or have sensitive skin should consult their herbalist or physician prior to selecting an aroma. Before use, always dilute in a carrier oil such as apricot kernel or sweet almond.

One day as I sat on an oak bench in our garden reading a book, I began really to look at the beautiful settee I was relaxing on. Grandpa and my father had made that bench by hand. The seat back was meticulously and intricately hand-carved with motifs of ancient Rome. The bench was an attractive centerpiece in our garden. On both sides Grandpa and my father had formed realistic oak leaf designs to pay reverence to this mighty tree.

Oak and walnut trees grew all around, towering above the bench and casting shadows that provided shade in the hot summer. It was my favorite place to think, dream, talk to Mother Nature, and read. It was a special place also to share my secrets with Grandma, my close girlfriends, and, of course, to meditate and communicate with the world of trees, birds, and azure sky.

Grandma used to say, "First of all, when you wake up in the morning, take a quick look at the sky . . . this endless spacious blue expanse . . . and you will feel comfortable."

The ancient Greeks believed that if you looked at the sky, even for a minute, it would cleanse your body, soul, and spirit and relieve you from "moral intoxication."

The garden bell, buoyed by the summer breeze, jingled a delicate melody. I was happy to be home again for summer vacation. A small shred of blue sky peeked through the branches of our old walnut trees as I read the works of the Russian poet and singer, Boulat Okoudjava. (You can hear him sing his heartfelt poems in Russian at http://www. russia-in-us.com/Music/Artists/index.html.

Here, sitting on this familiar and comforting bench, I began to daydream about the impact the changing seasons had on this spectacular garden. From spring to late fall, a profusion of flowers blossomed in Grandma's garden, but in winter under a blanket of snow, bulbs lay dormant and Grandma patiently waited for her favorite flowers to arrive. Finally the first messengers of awakening Nature arrived—delicate, milky-white snowdrops softly blowing in a tender breeze.

In "The Snowdrop" (1863) by Hans Christian Andersen, this spring flower was always wondering.

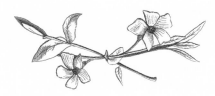

It was winter time; the air was cold, the wind was sharp, but within the closed doors it was warm and comfortable, and within the closed door lay the flower; it lay in the bulb under the snow-covered earth. One day rain fell. The drops penetrated through the snowy covering down into the earth, touched the flower bulb, and talked of the bright world above. Soon the Sunbeam pierced its way through the snow to the root, and within the root there was a stirring.

"Come in," said the Flower.

"I cannot," said the Sunbeam. "I am not strong enough to unlock the door! When the summer comes, I shall be strong!"

"When will it be summer?" asked the Flower, and she repeated this question each time a new sunbeam made its way down to her. But the summer was yet far distant. The snow still lay upon the ground, and there was a coat of ice on the water every night.

"What a long time it takes! What a long time it takes!" said the Flower. "I feel a stirring and striving within me; I must stretch myself, I must unlock the door, I must get out, and must nod a good morning to the summer, and a happy time that will be!"

In an old legend that Grandma breathed new life into, snow fell as Adam and Eve were banished from Paradise. There was no place for Eve to hide from the frost. Then several snowflakes transformed into beautiful flowers and offered her a sign of hope. From then on, the modest snowdrop was a symbol of hope.

White snowdrops rocked in the cradle of a light breeze. Each tiny flower, their white bell-shaped petals edged by the tiniest dab of lime green, shimmered in our garden. Grandma's flower of spring came to us from beneath the snow, a simple flower, carrying so much hope and joy for everyone.

Grandma cultivated in our garden only flowers that made good sense to her. She planted periwinkles, in spite of a common belief in Italy that the periwinkle is "the flower of the dead."

"So what?" she said. "My garden is not a garden without periwinkles. They bring happiness, as my garden brings relaxation."

The periwinkle is a symbol of everlasting life but is also considered by many to be a flower symbolizing jealousy. But Grandma did not think so and she told me a fairy tale about the periwinkle's little-known secret.

The periwinkle is one of the first flowers to blossom in the spring. Like the fragrant violet, it announces the coming spring, but the periwinkle was upset that people and the gods paid more attention to the violet than to it. However, the periwinkle's leaves and flowers are not less beautiful than that of the violet; only in fragrance does the violet surpass the periwinkle.

Once, when the goddess Flora came down to the earth in spring, she was charmed with the delicate smell of the violet. She caressed it and offered to make it taller, so it could tower over the other flowers, instead of smelling sweetly living discreetly in the shadows of other plants.

Suddenly a thin, whining voice sounded.

"Who is complaining?" Flora asked.

"It is me," replied the periwinkle.

"What do you want? Why are you crying?"

"I cry because you, the mother of flowers, don't notice me while at the same time you pour over the violet your graces and offer to make it better."

Flora looked at the little plant which she did not know at all or maybe she had just forgotten. Gods often cannot remember every single creature they have made. And so Flora asked, "What is your name?"

"I don't have a name yet," answered the periwinkle.

"In that case what do you wish for?"

"I wish to have a pleasant smell like the violet. Give it to me, Flora, and I will be very, very grateful."

"Unfortunately, that I cannot give you," replied Flora. "A plant receives this miraculous gift when it is the will of the Creator. It is given to a plant through the kiss of a genius appointed to guard it. You were born without a scent."

"Give me some kind of special gift that can make me equal to the violet. I am even similar to it in color, but everyone loves the violet, not me."

"Okay," agreed the goddess. "Blossom much longer than the violet. Blossom even then when the violet is long gone."

"Thank you, Flora. This is a great gift. Now when lovers try to find shady spots in gardens or parks and don't run into a violet, then maybe they will pay attention to me. They will take me and attach small bouquets of flowers to their chest near hearts beating with love."

"It can happen," responded the goddess.

"But I would like to ask you something else," continued the periwinkle. "Make my flowers larger than the violet's."

"As you wish. I can do that also. Let your flowers be larger than the violet's. The size does not indicate depth. Your looks say nothing about how intelligent you are."

Flora became irritated with the periwinkle's persistence and wanted to leave, but it seemed that the plant wasn't satisfied yet.

"What else do you want?" asked Flora. "You get a larger flower than the violet. You will blossom longer that it will. Isn't that enough?"

"No, Flora, since you are already so nice to me, then give me a name also, because without a name I am nothing."

Instead of becoming upset, Flora simply smiled.

"Okay, that's easy enough," she said. "You'll be named Pervinca from the Latin verb meaning *win* because no matter what, you always want to defeat your more modest and beautiful neighbor. Let your name be the expression of your jealous nature."

And from that time on the flower was called *periwinkle*.

There is a Ukrainian belief that a bouquet of periwinkles is a symbol of love and fidelity and those who plant periwinkles can be assured that their dreams will come true. In France there is a common notion that the demure periwinkle is the "witch's violet." Even so, during a recent trip to Switzerland, I noticed blue periwinkles encircling the monument of Jean-Jacques Rousseau, an eighteenth-century French writer and philosopher, on the tiny *Ile Rousseau* in Lake Geneva. The periwinkle was a favorite flower of Rousseau, and his first love, a French baroness Françoise-Louise de Warens, also called Madame de Warens. It was particularly special to Rousseau because it reminded him of the good years of his youth and the love that he lost.

Rousseau met her in 1728 on Palm Sunday, a moveable feast in the church calendar observed by Catholic, Orthodox, and Protestant Christians. This Sunday before Easter changed his life forever. Still a youth, just past boyhood, the kindhearted Madame de Warens hid Rousseau from Swiss authorities who were after him. He fell deeply in love with her and considered this the happiest time of his life. When they were traveling together from Chambéry (the capital of Savoy, France) to the countryside in Rhône-Alps, Madam de Warens saw a blue periwinkle in the bushes. She approached the flower and exclaimed, "Ah! *Voila de la pervenche en fleurs!*" ("This is a periwinkle blossoming!") Rousseau didn't respond to her exclamation, but that moment made a deep impression in his soul.

Many years passed, and as he walked with one of his friends on a picturesque mountainside near Neushâtel in Switzerland, he accidentally came upon the same flower. His happy past flashed before his eyes and in admiration he exclaimed, "Ah! *Voila de la pervenche en fleurs!*"

This exclamation returned many years after his happy travels with Françoise-Louise de Warens. Rousseau wrote about this in his autobiographical work, *Confessions*. When this book was first published and Parisians read this touching story, many visited the famous botanical garden, *Jardin des plantes* (Garden of Plants), to view the periwinkles there that were planted in Rousseau's honor.

The pert and pretty flowers also made an appearance in Hans Christian Andersen's fairy tale "Little Ida's Flowers" in 1835. The flowers that he wrote of loved grand balls where they merrily danced all night.

t was at one of those balls, that when the door to the room opened, a number of beautiful flowers danced in. Little Ida could not imagine where they had come from, unless they were flowers from the king's garden. First came two lovely roses wearing tiny golden crowns on their heads; these were the king and queen. Beautiful stocks and carnations followed, bowing to everyone present. They brought their own instruments with them. Large poppies and peonies had pea-shells, which they played and blew into them till they were quite red in the face. Bunches of blue hyacinths and the little white snowdrops jingled their bell-like flowers, as if they were real bells. Then came many more flowers: blue violets, purple heartsease, daisies, and lilies of the valley, and they all danced together and kissed one another. It was beautiful to behold."

So you see the small periwinkle is a flower of great magnitude after all. He is not so "sophisticated" as other beautiful flowers in Hans Christian Andersen's fairy tale which loved grand balls, but he is very cute and knows what he is doing, for sure.

D. Get a pet to fend off distress

Having a pet in the house can help us overcome bad stress. You will reap health benefits from keeping your loyal and responsive four-legged friends near you. American scientists discovered that people who have dogs live longer, happier lives. After observing patients who had suffered heart attacks, they concluded that owners of dogs recover four times faster than people without dogs. Why? Dogs provide their owners with unconditional love and daily walks outdoors in the fresh air, and they never argue with them. In addition, caring for a pet, whether cat or dog, fish, hamster, you name it, is an act of nurturing that gives as well as receives.

E. Stay intellectually active

If our lives are empty and we have nothing to do in our spare time, we become bored and mislabel the condition as stress. And indeed, being bored can lead to distress. The remedy for boredom is simple.

Stimulate yourself intellectually. Maintain a consistent process of self-improvement and you will find your life is full. Allow yourself to take time off from responsibilities and have fun! We can indulge our interests and satisfy our soul's starvation by going to the theater or enjoying a concert or an art exhibit. Choose what you like and make it part of your relaxation regime.

Good books are like good friends. Meet with people who share your reading interests. I know a group of women in Florida who meet once a week to read and critique a short story or book, or they may listen to music together or discuss the latest news events. By exchanging their ideas, they broaden their scope of interests and stimulate their intellect right there inside the four walls of their homes.

Exploring new impressions and knowledge can be like stashing treasures into a bottomless chest. Sometimes we have to give ourselves a gentle push past our inertia to satisfy our soul's desires. We can bring joy to our lives by engaging in simple pleasures like reading a good story or an uplifting article, going to a concert, or keeping a rendezvous with a friend, planting seeds or selecting flowers to fill a bouquet.

A Russian fable says that long, long ago before people existed on our planet, a green leaf sprouted from the earth. It stretched tall and stately to the sky, toward the sun, and blossomed as a lovely, crimson flower. And then another flower bloomed . . . and then another. Fields and mountainsides were painted in a wash of fragrance, texture, and color. In this way, beauty appeared in the world. The flowers evoked human emotions, thoughts, and words. These marvelous creations of Nature intermingled with our destinies, our traditions, and our lives.

Our house was always festively adorned with fresh flowers, either plucked from our bountiful garden or bestowed upon the family by Mama's thankful patients. She used to say, "Flowers have always given me the best feelings I know, and they remind me to be cheerful."

When the sunny days of my family's favorite season—summer—came to an end, a fog would shroud the meadows in the morning and we knew fall would soon be upon us. We felt an impending melancholy, yet a blue sky still smiled at us often and the forests still wore their multicolored attire. The earth wore a coverlet of fallen gold, scarlet, and indigo leaves. The last rose of summer, a smudge of crimson paint against a fading canvas, loomed in a corner of our yard. Luxurious white and purple chrysanthemums and pink asters rose up from the remaining soil.

Flowers bring beauty to our life, along with freshness and good feelings. They truly take away "the fall's melancholy"—our distress.

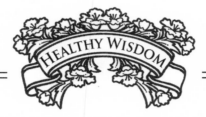

More than anything, I must have flowers, always, always.

—*Claude Monet (1840–1926), French impressionist painter*

Each flower is a soul opening out to nature.

—*Gerard de Nerval (1808–1855), French romantic writer*

He who is of a calm and happy nature will hardly feel the pressure of age,
but to him who is of an opposite disposition,
youth and age are equally a burden.

—*Plato,* The Republic

I never think of the future. It comes quickly enough.

—*Albert Einstein (1879–1955), German-born American physicist*

While there's life, there's hope.

—Cicero (106-43 B.C.), Roman orator, statesman, and philosopher

Life is as tedious as a twice-told tale.

—William Shakespeare (1564–1616), English playwright and poet

*Only the grasshoppers made a combined whirring, as if infuriated—
such an oppressive, unceasing, insipid, dry sound. It was appropriate
to the inhabiting midday heat as if literally by it, literally summoned by
it out of the sun-smelted earth.*

—Ivan Turgenev (1818–1883), Russian writer

*To analyze the charms of flowers is like dissecting music; it is one of those
things which it is far better to enjoy, than to attempt fully to understand.*

—Henry Theodore Tuckerman (1813–1871), American critic and writer

*What a pity flowers can utter no sound! A singing rose,
a whispering violet, a murmuring honeysuckle, oh, what a rare
and exquisite miracle would these be!*

—Henry Ward Beecher (1813–1887), American clergyman

*To me the meanest flower that blows can give thoughts
that do often lie too deep for tears.*

—William Wordsworth (1770–1850), English poet

A smooth sea never made a skillful mariner.

—English proverb

Chapter 11

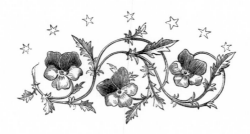

Trips to the Fairyland

Come in here. All my flowers would love to see you.

—*Grandma*

FACTS

Asthma is increasing in the United States and around the world. The prevalence of asthma around the world has doubled in the past 15 years.[33]

How many people have asthma in the United States?

- Approximately 24.7 million people in the United States have been diagnosed with asthma, with at least 7.7 million of them children under the age of 18.

- Asthma is the leading, serious, chronic illness among children in the United States.

Nearly 1 in 13 children in the United States has asthma, and this number is growing more rapidly in preschool-age children than in any other group.[34] The number of asthma-related visits to office-based physicians was 11.3 million in 2001.[35] The number of hospital emergency department visits connected with asthma attacks was 1.9 million in 2002.[36]

The Healthy People 2010 project reports the rate of asthma hospitalizations in children under age five is 45.6 per 10,000 and 12.5 per 10,000 for children five or over and adults. The goal is to reduce these rates.[37]

inkling bells outside my window woke me up in the middle of the night. I rose from my sound sleep, slid aside the vase on my windowsill filled with fragrant purple lilacs and sunny yellow tulips, and pushed open the window. As my vision adjusted to the darkness and shapes took form, I stood admiring the beautiful Fairyland in tones of shadowy indigo.

My grandma had inherited this land from my great-grandmother, when at 18 years old she married my grandfather. She called it her Dream Garden. Certainly it was enchanting under the light of the moon, in its slumbering, nocturnal state. Lilacs were in bloom and their sweet, pungent aroma permeated the cool night air. The bushes were heavy with luxuriant clusters of white and purple lilacs that opened widely their tiny star-shaped flowers. They rocked in unison, embraced by the gentle breeze. Spring, in all its glory, was upon this drowsy garden.

This stunningly beautiful place was only a small part of the original Fairyland, planted by my great-grandmother. My grandmother had followed in her steps and brought there her inspiration, joy, passion, skill, happiness, and a profound love of Nature. She was so proud of her accomplishments and always delighted in showing her garden.

"Come in here," she would say invitingly to our neighbors and friends. "All my flowers would love to see you. Show them your kind faces and they will smile at you."

The tinkling bells sounded louder, but they were not garden bells at all. The sounds came from a gracious nightingale, perched on the white lilac bush and singing a melodic song. I guessed that the aroma of the lilacs had intoxicated and inspired her to serenade all the living creatures, flowers, trees, and plants throughout the night.

I remember many years ago, watching my grandma sitting in her favorite rocking chair beneath a bush of fragrant lilac. Who knows? Perhaps while relaxing in her garden during these quiet hours of the evening, she was thinking how blessed she was with her happy family life and good health, how thankful she was that she had been so beautiful in her youth that many boys had chased her, admiring her good looks. On the old pictures that she kept carefully in the family album, she looked small with a healthy, thick mane of black, shiny hair. Her huge blue eyes shone like the stars under a navy umbrella of the night sky.

She liked to tell me about her teenage years, especially when she was 18. According to her, men approached women in a careful and gentle manner then. A manner of respect was a centuries-old tradition. When a young man approached a young woman, instead of leading with questions such as "What is your name? How are you?" they would present themselves with great reverence to the woman and say, "Please allow me to introduce myself. May I kiss your hand, *mademoiselle*?"

This tradition was based on human dignity and a show of respect from a young man to a young woman. This question revealed a noble intention to make a first connection; a curious, sincere interest; and *attraction* at first sight, not *love* at first sight.

It was once upon a time when my grandma sat in our Dream Garden with a handsome young man and heard the sweetest music to her ears—his first confession of love for her. As you might guess, the young man was my grandfather. He was a quiet, but ambitious and hard-working man. Later, with great motivational support from my grandmother, he created his "kingdom" of vineyards and orchards. They sat many, many times there during the long, balmy evenings of late spring, discussing plans for their future while dreaming in the Dream Garden. They looked in unison at the starry sky through tiny white lilac flowers, observing the movement of the clouds and planets, which witnessed silently their love and trust for each other, their ringing laughter and ecstatic kisses.

I recently revisited our Dream Garden and found it is still as much alive as it was many years ago. Other people—strangers to me—live there now, but the nightingale's soprano trill still fills the garden all night long until dawn and the air is still rich with the aroma of lilacs.

Nastoykas, with lilac flowers and buds from gardens like ours, are successfully used in folk medicine to treat rheumatism, osteoporosis (accumulation of salt in joints), podagra (inflammation of the feet), and heel spurs. Before I mention natural treatments for asthma, I want to tell you a little bit about how small, gracious, and fragrant lilacs can be effective healers in different sicknesses.

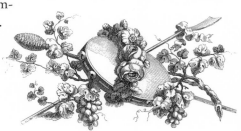

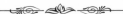

 1. Make Lilac Vodka. Add ¼ cup lilac flowers and crushed buds to one cup alcohol or vodka. Let steep for 8–10 days in a glass jar in a dark place at room temperature. Take 20–30 drops of lilac/alcohol nastoyka or 50 drops of lilac/vodka three times a day.

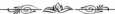

 2. Add 1 tablespoon dried lilac flowers to five ounces alcohol at 40 degrees. Let steep for eight to ten days in a glass gar with close-fitting lid. Take 30 drops two to three times a day.

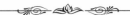

 3. Soak a cheesecloth in the same nastoyka (#2) and rub painful parts or make a compress and apply where necessary for the treatment of rheumatism, salt deposit in joints, or knee spur.

Lilac is effective for external treatment. Lilac bushes blossom in May and those who practice folk medicine gather the buds shortly after they bloom.

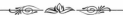

 4. Fill three quart glass jars with fresh lilac blossoms. Add enough lamp oil or turpentine oil to cover. Cover with a lid and allow to infuse for two weeks in a dark place. Then rub this mixture one to two times a day into painful joints until they are red. Then wrap this part of the body with a flannel fabric or wool scarf to keep it warm for one hour. Your pain will disappear.

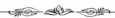

n ancient Greek legend tells that Pan (called Faunas by the Romans), the god of forests and meadows, nature and the universe, fell hopelessly in love with a nymph named Syringe. This is the way that I remember the tale, after years of hearing it from Grandma and Mama and many more years of sharing it with my own children.

Pan was strolling through a lush, sylvan setting when he met a river nymph named Syringe, known for heralding the dawn of a new day. Pan was so spellbound by Syringe's graciousness and beauty that he instantly fell in love with her and he lost sight of everything for which he was responsible.

He was so obviously struck by her that she became frightened of him and ran away. Pan pursued her, all the while trying to assure here that his intentions were noble. The nymph did not reply, but instead transformed into a fragrant bush with delicate purple flowers. Devastated, Pan fell to his knees and wept for many hours, soaking the earth under the lilac bush.

The next day when Pan revisited the bush, he saw that it was stronger and larger and that a profusion of new blossoms had appeared overnight. Its branches were heavy with clusters of sweet-scented lilacs. He was captured by the beauty of the bush and from somewhere he clearly heard the sound of a woman's voice, pure and delicate as the lilacs, "I know now, Pan, that your love for me was true and strong. Your bittersweet tears have provided sustenance for me, given me strength and enduring beauty. I promise you that in return for your suffering, I will love all as you have loved me by providing them my secrets of abundant health and beauty."

Pan was inspired by Syringe's courage and benevolence and he too became overwhelmed by the power of pure love. He proclaimed loudly to all creatures of the forest, "At his very moment the lilac bush will take the Latin name of Syringe and she will bestow her kindness on anyone who happens upon her. Her beauty and aroma will delight the senses and her medicine will heal the body."

Pan ceased to roam the forest groves in grief. Instead his inward grief manifested itself as an outward expression of the love he would forever have for Syringe and he began to perform many kind deeds for all he met.

Lilac takes its name from the Greek word *syrinx*, which means a tube. Shepherds have cut pipes or flutes from the wood of the lilac bush. So perhaps when you visit Alpine meadows or those of the Appalachians, Rockies, Carpathian, Caucasus Mountains, or others, you may hear and enjoy the beautiful and unforgettable sound of a lilac pipe played by shepherds. In Russia the lilac is known as *synel* and *cyren* from the word *ciniy* (blue). In Russia the lilac grows in purple and white and sky blue, pale pink, golden yellow, and burnt orange.

Infuse a bit of Fairyland into your own backyard by planting a lilac bush there. Enjoy its vibrant beauty and tantalizing fragrance. Each year the month of May will bring fresh blossoms to the bush. Cut fresh purple or blue clusters and combine them with yellow tulips. White lilac flowers blend well with pink peonies. Arrange them in a big crystal vase as a centerpiece of a table or windowsill to bring the beauty of your garden indoors. It will refresh the air and bring Nature into your life. **Remember** that cut lilacs do not enjoy other "neighbors" in a vase, so this colorful combination is good only for a short time.

Another legend, revised somewhat by its numerous repetitions throughout our family, tells us about the origin of lilacs.

Many years ago lilacs came into being when Spring washed away the snow from the meadows and the golden sun rose to the top of the cerulean sky. The sun was accompanied by a rainbow when it began its movement above the earth. Spring, gathering colors to toss upon the earth, decided to mix the sun's beams with the rainbow's rays as it continued to move from south to north and then threw the color mixture to earth. Everywhere the vibrant mixture of rays and beams fell, flowers blossomed in sky-blue, navy, yellow, orange, and red.

When Spring reached the north, she had only purple and white remaining, but there the weather was still very cold in the Scandinavian countries, including Sweden, Norway, Holland, and Denmark. However Spring was wise and tossed the purple color to earth where it became small, shiny star-shaped flowers. Spring then sprinkled the white generously above the earth. It fell like powdered sugar over the small, bare bushes, creating a myriad of delicate lilac flowers.

Beautiful fragrant lilac, coming to us from legends into our Dream Gardens, is a beautiful reminder that every year in May, spring will arrive in full prosperity and together with Nature awaken us from a long winter's nap. Spring will dress the trees and bushes with buds and bright, young green leaves. Then spring will throw the seeds of admiration and wonder into the forests' glades and meadows, and very soon in summer they will blossom into a rainbow of flawless flowers.

Each flower will appear in all its magnificence, emitting its own unique fragrance, coming from the glowing and consistently moving world of Nature. Come to this fantastic meadow of flowers! Breathe the fresh air! This beautiful Fairyland is created for us by Nature. Relax and allow new energy to pour into your body. Your eyes will brighten. Your mind will become clear. Positive emotions and bright thinking will enlighten you. The stress of day-to-day life will fall away. Your healthy spirit will return and you will be ready to climb mountains.

I believe that good energy and positive thinking are all pervasive. A healthy life is based on these two powerful factors. Positive energy and positive thinking combine to become a beautiful airy lace, knit with our thoughts and bio-currents. Throughout many years I have observed that when the weather is cloudy and the sun hides behind the heavens, some people have little energy since the sun passes us its creative life force. Without it, we are weak.

Try this: When you commune with Nature, relax and enjoy how the flowers and trees send you their messages and signals. Let your heart and soul be open and receptive to the feeling of a strong emotional union with Nature. Gently release any thoughts that enter your mind. Rest and relax. Breathe deeply and smell the fragrance of the flowers. You will feel refreshed and rejuvenated and ready to face another day of responsibilities and decisions with a clear head.

If instead you feel unhappy or fatigued:

---

 5. Make fresh pomegranate juice, add one teaspoon honey to eight ounces, and drink it.

---

 6. Make a cup of green tea. Mix it with white or black tea and pour in it several drops of pomegranate juice instead of lemon. It will lift the spirit and soften the heart. It will promote energy, refresh the body, and clear sensitivity formed by toxic negativity.

Grandma taught me this one:

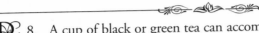

 7. Make a special egg-milk drink to combat fatigue. Stir one raw yolk (of an organic egg) in a cup with hot milk. Add one teaspoon honey and mix well. Drink slowly and enjoy.

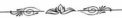

 8. A cup of black or green tea can accompany the following remedy, which is adopted from Tibetan medicine. It is a natural treatment for fatigue and headaches and for strengthening the heart. Mix and eat one ounce walnuts, 1½ ounces cheese (Muenster, Mozzarella, Swiss, White American, or Smoked Gouda), and 1½ ounces raisins.

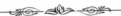

 9. Add one fresh quince or a teaspoon of quince preserves to your green, black, or black currant tea. A quince gives a special taste and delicate aroma like no other ingredient.

We used many plants from our Dream Garden—our family Fairyland—as natural medicines, libations, tinctures, nastoykas, decoctions, balsams, syrups, and medicinal herbal teas. Mother Nature provides us with special plants to treat a variety of illnesses.

- The oak tree stands out as a healing remedy for people suffering with high blood pressure.

- Coniferous trees and bushes are healers for people with tuberculosis.

- Poplar, hawthorn, eucalyptus, lilac, and bay serve people with cardiovascular diseases.

- Linden and oregano plants help people with respiratory ailments.

- Lavender, mint, and geranium heal people with neuroses and other dysfunctions of the central nervous system.

For many centuries humans have developed a close contact with the world of plants, but even so we have strayed far from Mother Nature. Increasingly, as time goes by, we lose this valuable connection with the perfect world of trees and herbs. More and more our precious rain forests with their abundance of healing plants are being destroyed by the bulldozer's bite. Each day we inhale the toxic fumes of gasoline and other chemicals and the living aromas of natural plants disappear from our homes in exchange for the so-called beauty of silk flowers.

Less and less we breathe in the marvelous natural scents of trees, earth, and snow that bring us health and energy. When I was a little girl, we always had plants such as eucalyptus, aloe, or a branch of a coniferous tree in our home. Near our house grew a proud pine which we knew always gave us energy and oxygen. In our garden Grandma cultivated mint and lavender; the modest, but fragrant chamomile; oregano; and King's clover or thyme. She sewed by hand small pretty cotton sachets, which she stuffed with fresh herbs and hung in our closets and on nails throughout our house. They emitted an intense aroma that made us feel as if we had come to change our clothes in a fragrant garden.

Over many years I've observed that our memory of smells (our olfactory sense) is much stronger than our visual or auditory (acoustic) memory. Even now, as I am writing this book, I clearly recall the familiar fragrance of chamomile from my childhood. Its aroma reminds me of many events in the past. When I hold a sprig of chamomile in my hand, I breathe in its aroma and instantly recall my brightest memories and become happy and content.

I realize why this happens. Our sense of smell is connected closely to the part of our brain that rules our memory and our emotions. Different aromas influence the activity in our internal systems. Our brain's limbic system, at the root of the cerebral cortex, releases neurotransmitters (messengers within our body), including endorphins and encephalin, both of which diminish pain and promote an overall sense of well-being; serotonin, which relaxes us; and adrenaline, which keeps us stimulated and alert. Aromas have the ability to call up positive and negative emotions.

Two famous ancient doctors, Hippocrates and Avicenna, used aromas to treat headaches and sleeplessness. Using herbal aromas as remedies, which is what we now call aromatherapy, has been popular for many centuries in ancient Russia, China, and Egypt. For instance, one ancient Chinese doctor discovered that the smell of dried chrysanthemum, lily, nutmeg, and sandalwood helps lower high blood pressure and heal sleep disorders and some respiratory ailments.

Lily can treat skin disorders too. An ancient French remedy recommends:

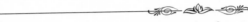

 10. Cook the bulb of a lily until soft, mix it with honey, and apply to your face. It will smooth wrinkles, diminish facial spots, and soothe herpes and eczema.

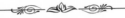

Chrysanthemum was brought to Europe in 1676 from Japan, the land of the rising sun. In Japan this flower heralds fall and is a symbol of the sun and the Japanese nation. For a long time the image of a chrysanthemum was sacred in Japan. Only the emperor and his family members had the right to wear clothing imprinted with the chrysanthemum design. The legend about Japan's origin came from the magical characteristics of this last flower of the year, which appears during the initial days of fall. It explains why these beautiful, feathery white flowers are as attractive as the first autumn frost, breathing on us the first fresh air that allows Nature to fall asleep for a long winter's dream.

Here is another tale that was popular in our household. Again it has been revised over several interpretations and reiterations and is formed now in our own words.

In ancient times a cruel emperor ruled China. One day he was told that a marvelous healing flower grew on an island near China. He was told that a magical Elixir of Life could be prepared from the oils of this flower, but only people with a kind heart and noble intentions could pick this flower. The emperor and all his court had committed so many sins in their lives that they decided not to take the risk and instead they sent three hundred young men and women to the island to pick these chrysanthemums. The young people were instantly charmed by the beauty of the island, refused to obey his orders, and never returned with the chrysanthemums. They had fallen in love with this island and founded there—in the land of the rising sun—a new country, Japan.

According to Italian legend, chrysanthemums first appeared from paper flowers that a poor woman had used to decorate the grave of her son. The next morning she visited his grave with new paper flowers but was greatly amazed to see that the paper flowers she had left before had magically transformed. They had sprouted and become beautiful fresh white chrysanthemums.

Chrysanthemums became a symbol of chastity, purity, innocence, and fidelity. Thus, if you fall in love in the frosty fall, give your beloved a lovely bouquet of white chrysanthemums generously given to us by Nature.

In 4,000 B.C. Egyptians distilled the essential oils of plants such as coriander, cinnamon, and cedar for use in cosmetics, medicine, and mummification.

For centuries in Russia it was popular to treat sleeplessness by using a pillow filled with dried hops, which acts as a sedative on the central nervous system. It slows the metabolism and brings about a sound sleep. Dried hops used in pillows for sleeplessness should be replaced every two to three months because aged strobiles (cones) may produce a counter effect and stimulate instead of sedate.

Aromas of geranium, laurel noble, and rosemary can have a soothing effect on people with nervous disorders, shortness of breath, poor circulation, and chronic bronchitis. I know that those particular fragrances were tremendously helpful to Mama in overcoming her own health problems.

One of the bright impressions in my childhood was a trip to a real Fairyland. Once in the summer I spent my vacation with Mama in Crimea, a beautiful resort located on the shores of the Black Sea. At that time Mama had severe problems with allergic bronchial asthma. She prescribed for herself a special treatment using the aromas of certain plants, which we found in an enchanting place known as Karasan in Crimea.

A park in the Crimean sanatorium, created in the nineteenth century during the reign of a Russian czar, was divided into five areas with each area planted with herbs, flowers, and trees having aromas which influenced particular human conditions. Although their gardens differed from one another, each shared a common goal—to be useful as healing plants. These sections were:

- laurel—to stop spasms
- coniferous trees—to increase energy and lung capacity
- rose and lavender—to calm the nervous system
- jasmine—to stimulate the brain
- rosemary—to combat chronic respiratory diseases

The area Mama visited most was lush with rosemary. That hot summer we spent many hours in this memorable old park with deep shadows, cool shade, and incredible fresh air thick with the scents of herbs and flowers.

So what is bronchial asthma that Mama suffered from? It is a chronic disease of the respiratory system. Its symptoms include periodic asthmatic's fits of various intensity and duration. An episode can last from several hours to several days. An attack is characterized by bronchi spasms, swelling of the mucous membranes, and an accumulation of mucus, which begins to exude.

Usually asthma attacks appear suddenly at night, when we sleep peacefully. We experience difficulty in breathing, swelling of the chest cavity, and a feeling of stifled breath. There may be a whistling to the breath, the face may become blue, and the blood vessels in the neck may swell. At the end of an asthmatic attack, the volume of mucus increases and is easily expelled.

In some cases those affected by asthma experience "prolonged asthma." In this condition it can take days and hours to stop an asthmatic fit, but this can happen only if the sickness was not diagnosed initially and treated properly.

What to do externally to ease a sudden asthmatic attack?

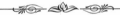

 11. Open windows to allow fresh air into the room. Place both hands and feet in a tub of hot water to which a pinch of mustard powder has been added. Rub your chest with a towel or other soft fabric, which has been soaked in cold water to which vinegar and iodized salt have been added.

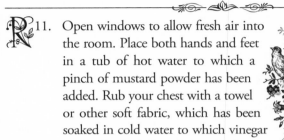

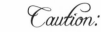 *Caution:*

People with pulmonary diseases cannot use this method. Consult your physician.

 12. Massage the upper part of your body from your head down to the top of your chest and back, using a nutritious crème, talc, or rice powder.

If an unexpected, sudden attack occurs:

 13. Inhale an ammonia capsule, typically used for fainting.

 14. Apply mustard plasters to the calves.

 15. Suck on ice chips.

 16. Drink warm finely-ground barley coffee.

17. Inhale the aroma of fresh pine to increase lung capacity and promote energy.

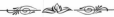

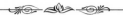

 18. Inhale the aroma of laurel leaves to help diminish spasms.

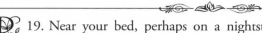

 19. Near your bed, perhaps on a nightstand, place a small bowl filled with liquid ammonia to cleanse the air. This is particularly helpful if you live in a hot, tropical climate and cannot open the windows.

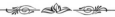

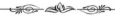 20. Keep a geranium plant in your house to cleanse the air of dust and bacteria.

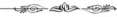

 21. Burn the dry leaves of coltsfoot and breathe in its healing smoke. It is a soothing expectorant.

 22. Mix ¼ cup dry wine (Riesling, Chardonnay) with a pinch of baking soda. Drink it to promote mucus dilution during an asthmatic fit.

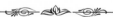

 23. Place two to three hot, boiled potatoes in a bowl. Cover your head with a thick towel and inhale the medicinal steam to soothe spasms and ease breathing.

24. Prepare hot red bilberry tea, using one tablespoon fresh or dried berries and leaves in one cup boiling water. Steep 15 minutes and drink during an asthmatic fit. Lie down in bed and cover yourself with a blanket to preserve the warmth of the red bilberry tea in your system. Use this simple remedy in combination with potato medicinal steam (#23). These two methods are effective natural healers in your defense against asthmatic attacks. After at least one month of treatments in this manner, the attacks are likely to occur with less frequency.

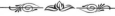

For less intense asthmatic episodes, treatment can be limited to drinking hot red bilberry tea only.

25. Take a pine bath. Place two cups pine needles, cones, and twigs in a pot with two quarts cold water. Boil 30 minutes. Cover pot and infuse for 10–12 hours. A pine bath rejuvenates and increases the supply of energy not only in bronchial asthma, but in other respiratory illnesses.

 26. Pine steam, saturated with essential oil, heals mucous membranes. Add 25–30 drops of essential pine oil (made from pine needles only) in two cups hot water and inhale pine steam.

 27. Honey inhalation. Mix one tablespoon honey with two cups hot distilled water. Pour one tablespoon honey water into an inhaler and breathe in for 15–20 minutes. Use this only if you are not allergic to honey.

Just a reminder. As you know, the main task in treating bronchial asthma is "to liberate" or to cleanse bronchi of mucus, which promotes asthmatic attacks. Help yourself with pleasant treatments, such as:

 28. Walking in the pine woods.

 29. Drinking warm mineral water. It contains alkali, which helps to cleanse phlegm from the bronchi.

 30. Getting proper exercise to cleanse lungs and bronchi.

The above three treatments can be used for those with cardiovascular diseases. What can we do internally to treat asthma in a natural way?

 31. Grate 3½ ounces horseradish root, add juice of two lemons, and mix well to create a thick syrup. Take ½ teaspoon twice daily for one month. Refrigerate for no more than 7–10 days.

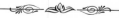

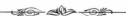

 32. Take two tablespoons honey twice daily if you are not allergic to it.

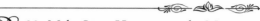

 33. Make Juicy Honey remedy. Mix one cup fresh carrot juice, one cup horseradish juice, and the juice of one lemon. Add one cup honey, mix well, and pour into a glass jar. Take one teaspoon one hour before meals three times a day. Refrigerate the remaining mixture. The course of treatment is two months.

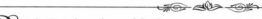

 34. Drink a glass of fresh grape juice daily to treat bronchial asthma and respiratory problems.

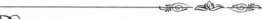

 35. Place one tablespoon anise seeds into a pot with one cup boiling water. Cook seeds 15 minutes. Take ¼ cup four times a day before meals.

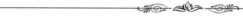

 36. To two tablespoons of diced turnip roots, add two cups of boiling water. Boil 15 minutes. Strain and drink ¼ cup four times a day or one cup before bed.

 37. Boil two to three turnips in one quart of water for five minutes. Drink ⅓ cup three times a day.

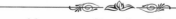

 38. Infuse two tablespoons of wild marjoram in two cups of boiling water for 15 minutes. Strain and divide the infusion into three portions. Take three times a day 30 minutes before meals as an expectorant.

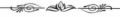

39. Add three tablespoons of hawthorn berries to one cup of boiling water. Infuse for 30 minutes and drink one cup three times a day for asthma attacks.

40. Add two tablespoons of fresh or dried wild strawberry leaves to two cups of boiling water. Infuse for 15 minutes. Drink one cup daily for asthma attacks as a cleansing diuretic.

 41. Add one tablespoon of dry or fresh plantain leaves to one cup of boiling water. Infuse for 15 minutes. Strain and take one tablespoon four times a day as a cough suppressant.

 42. Mix together one tablespoon each elder, plantain, heartsease, and sundew (*Drosera rotundifolia*) dry or fresh flowers. Place one tablespoon of the mixture and one cup of cold water into a pot. Infuse for two hours, then bring to a boil for five minutes. Cool, strain, and take ⅓ cup three times a day for one month.

 43. Following the above method (#42), mix together one tablespoon each of elder and young willow bark and two tablespoons each of anise seeds and rose hips.

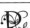 44. Mix three tablespoons raspberry root with one pint water and cook slowly for 15 minutes. Cool and take two to three tablespoons four times a day.

 45. Mix together one tablespoon each of thyme, pine buds, anise seeds, and fennel. Place one tablespoon of this mixture into a pot. Add one cup spring water. Place the pot inside a bigger one filled with hot water and warm up for 15 minutes in a "steaming bath." Take ¼ cup three to four times a day.

 46. Mix one tablespoon each of fennel, licorice root, pine buds, thyme, and anise seeds. Place two tablespoons of herbal mixture into one cup of water. Warm up in "a steaming bath" (as in #44) for 15 minutes. Infuse for 30 minutes, strain. You should have one-half of the liquid remaining. Add boiled water to make one cup. Take ⅓ cup three to four times a day.

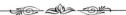

 47. Mix one tablespoon each of calendula flowers, diced wild marjoram root, diced licorice root, plantain, anise seeds, and heartsease leaves. The method of preparation is the same as in #45.

 48. Make "Mashed Onions." Peel and dice 20 small "baby" onions, add one pint boiling water, and infuse for 10 minutes until onions are soft. Add one cup olive oil and mix well to make a puree. Take one tablespoon of "Mashed Onions" before breakfast.

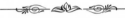

 49. Make garlic butter. Grate five to seven large garlic cloves and mix well with three ounces salted, organic butter. Spread on a slice of rye bread or add to pasta or mashed potatoes. It is an effective bactericidal and soothing natural healer for bronchial asthma and respiratory diseases.

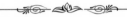

 50. Make "Drunk Aloe" balsam. Mix ½ pound fresh aloe leaves and one pint Cahors (Port) wine with 12 ounces honey. You can purchase an aloe plant in a nursery or purchase the leaves in some specialty supermarkets. Place an aloe plant on a windowsill in your house or on a porch. Do not water aloe for two weeks. Aloe can live without water for a long time—aloe's nickname is "a century old." After two weeks cut the leaves; clean dust from them but do not wash them. Dice the leaves and place in a glass jar. Add wine and honey, mix well, and infuse for eight to nine days in a cool place. Strain and take one tablespoon three times a day for the first two days. Then take one teaspoon three times a day until this medicinal balsam is gone. Aloe is an effective healer for bronchial asthma, pneumonia, and tuberculosis.

Caution:

Do not use aloe in the presence of uterine bleeding because it promotes a rush of blood to internal organs.

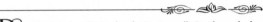

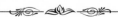

51. My mother effectively treated bronchial asthma with the common ginger plant. Here is her nastoyka treatment. Wash ½ pound ginger, peel, and grate. Place it into a glass jar and add vodka to cover. Infuse it in a warm place indoors or outside in the summer. Shake the jar occasionally and when the liquid turns an amber color, strain and allow it to settle. Dissolve one teaspoon in ½ cup spring water and take twice daily, after breakfast and after dinner. Continue for three days, stop for three days, and then resume your treatment, following this schedule. **Remember**: When you take the ginger nastoyka remedy, do not consume meat. Also take a warm foot bath before bed.

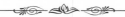

Aromatherapy, the science of inhaling plant extracts as a healing process, is an ancient practice. In this century we have many new ways to enjoy this art. We can bathe in essential oils, add them to pure base oils to create massage lotions, burn them in aroma lamps, or heat them in light bulb rings to scent the room and create a soothing atmosphere. With the wide range of essential oils available to us, we may use various essences to suit our needs and moods.

After years of research and experimentation, Swiss scientists have found that the most aromatic compound is found in grapefruit. It is so concentrated that a very small amount added to 250 gallons of water brings about an appreciable fruit scent.

For centuries, in ancient Russia, folk medicine practitioners successfully treated patients with aromatherapy. They were guided by practical considerations and their intuition. Seventeenth-century Russian books, carefully archived under seven seals, contain information about special wooden chambers, like mini bath houses called *chepuchines,* in which medicinal plants were steamed.

This method of treatment was known as *chepuchine* sitting. Those suffering from colds, rheumatism, infections, and other ailments sat in these baths and inhaled the medicinal and aromatic vapors of the steaming plants.

People in the Caucasus Mountains (Georgia, Armenia, the republics of the former Soviet Union) traditionally would wear a bulb of garlic around their neck as a talisman to prevent disease. The Caucasus Mountain range is also the famed "longevity belt," which attracted worldwide notice in the late 1960s. News reporters, scientists, and gerontologists were among those who trekked up the green, idyllic mountainsides, abundant in apples, potatoes, and flower and vegetable gardens, at an altitude of around a thousand feet above sea level, to research the villagers who lived there. The region was reported to be unusually populated with people who lived long lives, often far beyond 100 years—some were said to be as old as 110 to 140.

Shirali Mislimov was one man who lived in Azerbaijan who was reputed to be 168 at the time of his death in 1973! Diet and exercise are believed to be contributing factors to the population's longevity. I wonder if scientists also considered contributions made by the fragrant aromas of the villagers' lush mountain gardens, their tea fields, the sea, the fresh mountain air . . . .

In other ancient European countries and Russia, people used to burn branches of juniper during epidemics of disease. We can use it in this century during epidemics of flu.

People in the Ukraine use thyme to disinfect their homes from contagious diseases. For centuries, Ukrainians have filled mattresses with thyme and scattered this herb on their floors to freshen the air in their homes.

American Indians burn bundles of sage and juniper to purify their environment. In fact, the ritual is no longer confined to a specific culture and today is a popular purification process in the Western and Southwestern United States. In ancient India and China the aroma of lotus saved thousands of people from infectious diseases and the Black Death plague.

In my childhood home, we followed a tradition in the fall of washing all of our woolen rugs with pine soap. Grandma had made the rugs by hand. We rinsed them in salt water and allowed them to dry outside on a windy, sunny day. The air in our house was then refreshed with the aroma of pine until the following autumn. The scent was beneficial to the health of our lungs, throat, and bronchi.

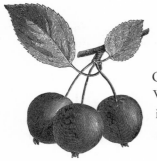

Please remember that natural, medicinal plants have strong disinfectant properties. They are tireless fighters in the bacterial "battlefield."

There are 35,000 microbes in one cubic yard of air. Our immune system must work hard to neutralize them. We should practice a regular exercise regime incorporating such aerobic activities as walking and jogging. Our use of essential plant oils with their bactericidal shields can then do a better job for our well-being.

Other valuable essential oils are derived from valerian, mint, fennel, anise, rose, lavender, and sage—most of which are also common culinary herbs. Please remember that essential oils are just that—the pure essence of the plant from which they are extracted. So-called blended oils which contain synthetic additives or synthetic oils should not be used for healing or to promote good health.

Essential oils can be expensive, as it often takes an vast amount of plants to produce a small amount of oil. For example, it takes 10,000 pounds of jasmine flowers to produce one pound of oil. Please insist on pure essential oils for your health.

Turn your house into a Fairyland every season of the year. Create your own health resort to heal your mind, body, and spirit. In winter, when the skin is especially dry, it is helpful to take warm, relaxing, and healing baths. Fill your bathtub with warm water. Pour ½ cup of vinegar and 25-30 drops of lavender oil and enjoy your way to relaxation.

Winter was never one of my favorite seasons, but one slow-moving, cold evening during a long winter I was determined to find something good in the bad. The snowflakes sparkled like diamonds and whirled slowly to earth in the cold air. They covered the ground with a fluffy and splendid blanket, knit with millions of beautiful radiant sequins. I was walking home from school. The brilliant, glistening white snow crunched under my feet. The air was fresh and crisp. A powerful north wind roared ferociously and brutally pounded the glass windows and wooden shutters of the houses. Our house stood up strong against the furious windy winter attack, thanks to the tall giant pines, oaks, and huge walnuts that buffered it. The trees squealed pitifully but stood strong and proud, fighting the cold demon bravely like the most courageous soldiers in the snowy battlefield.

I ran the last 10 steps until I was finally inside the house. There it was warm and cozy. Inside was the aroma of lilac and lavender and Papa played Peter Tchaikovsky's "The Seasons" on the piano in our *gostinaya* (a family room). The aroma of lilac flowed from a slick, purple candle, homemade in Grandma's "laboratory." As it slowly burned down, it cried fragrant lilac tears, drop by drop, falling onto a shiny silver plate in rhythm to the magnificent Tchaikovsky's summer part of "The Seasons"—"Barcarolle." I knew that Papa missed summer too.

Birch logs snapped and crackled in the fireplace, throwing sparks of the golden amber tongues of fire. The flames danced and curled wildly, but their show wasn't contained to the fireplace. They threw their shadows on the far side of the room, where their pale yellow and tangerine reflections trembled on the dark wall.

I felt peaceful and comfortable there. The warm atmosphere always made me feel cozy. I loved to read a good book there or daydream about mysterious places. I imagined flights on a magic carpet. I dreamed about an adventurous voyage on a "flying vessel" set to explore far away countries and discover new lands. It was my winter "Dream Garden" filled with books instead of plants. This memory is often brought back to me by the aromas of lilac, lavender, and burning birch and the sounds of Tchaikovsky's unforgettable music.

We had thousands of books in our home library. Reading was one of my favorite pastimes, especially in winter. We didn't have computers and computer games when I was growing up. We didn't have television broadcasts with boring, upsetting news and undelivered promises by politicians. It could never have substituted or competed anyway with the world of classic literature and music.

I savored the time I had to read masterpieces of literature, created by talented people throughout the world through the centuries. I convinced myself that the books would substitute successfully in the wintertime for all the fine, soft-petaled spring flowers; the bounty of sweet-smelling summer blossoms and herbs, their scents made stronger by the heat of the summer sun.

I imagined that the books I held in my hands were paper flowers, blooming with brilliant human thoughts, so I developed a "strange" habit. It amazes me now how dedicated I was to reading and how I read each book voraciously as if I were a starving peasant with an insatiable appetite, gobbling down each word as if it were my last bit of bread, my last drop of honey. I read volume after volume of Jules Vern's science fiction, Alexander Dumas' novels, and James Fennimore Cooper's colorful adventures. I devoured the works of Leo Tolstoy, Anton Chekhov, Fyodor Dostoyevsky, Honore de Balzak, Gustave Flaubert, Theodore Dreiser's dramas, Dante Alighieri, William Shakespeare's tragedies, and Walt Whitman's poems. It was a feeding frenzy. I never stopped reading an author's collection. I read volume after volume until I finished all of them. It was my passion. Reading was what I most hungered for in my life. I read all of their works, including the epistle genre: the letters they wrote to loved ones, friends, and other writers.

With all the tomes of literature at my fingertips, it was hard to say what I loved most, but I have to admit that my favorite books—even now—are unforgettable folktales and fairy tales from around the world. I had heard plenty of them from Grandma and I fell in love with these anthologies and will hold them dear to my heart for the rest of my life because these tales are good and wise. They reflect our real life, and they are a bright example of intelligent human thought. They became for me a window to the world and a brilliant tool with which to learn about it. After all, these beautiful stories came to me from the Fairyland, the mystical, magical land of fairies.

I learned a lot from fairy tales told by Dutch storyteller Hans Christian Andersen. I read almost all of them. Sometimes I explore his storehouse even now, and I find always there a mix of fantasy and true-life experience. I am full of wonder. I have learned about destiny, and I admire the noble actions of his heroes. I find I effortlessly float into his fairy tales and transcend this real life and all at once I am a character in another realm.

Our big candle shone with a small orange fire and quietly burned down, marking time by growing smaller, dropping purple tears, sharing the lovely ambiance of which it was a part with all of us in the room, its heady fragrance of lilac intoxicating us. Very soon this flower would celebrate spring in Grandma's Dream Garden, but winter was still upon us and so I nestled comfortably into a chair and read Hans Christian Andersen's "The Candles," a beautiful fairy tale written in 1870.

There was once a big wax candle which knew its own importance quite well. "I am born of wax and molded in a shape," it said. "I give better light and burn longer than other candles. My place is in a chandelier or on a silver candlestick!"

"That must be a lovely existence!" said the tallow candle. "I am only made of tallow, but I comfort myself with the thought that it is always a little better than being a farthing dip: That is only dipped twice, and I am dipped eight times, to get my proper thickness. I am content! It is certainly finer and more fortunate to be born of wax instead of tallow, but one does not settle one's own place in this world. You are placed in the big room in the glass chandelier, I remain in the kitchen, but that is also a good place; from there the whole house gets its food."

"But there is something which is more important than food," said the wax-candle. "Society! To see it shine, and to shine oneself! There is a ball this evening and soon I and all my family will be fetched."

Scarcely was the word spoken, when all the wax-candles were fetched, but the tallow candle also went with them. The lady herself took it in her dainty hand, and carried it out to the kitchen: a little boy stood there with a basket, which was filled with potatoes; two or three apples also found their way there. The good lady gave all this to the poor boy.

"There is a candle for you as well, my little friend," said she. "Your mother sits and works till late in the night; she can use it!"

The little daughter of the house stood close by, and when she heard the words 'late in the night,' she said with great delight, "I also shall stay up till late in the night! We shall have a ball, and I shall wear my big red sash!"

How her face shone with joy! No wax candle can shine like two childish eyes!

"That is a blessing to see," thought the tallow candle; "I shall never forget it and I shall certainly never see it again."

Maybe the tallow candle referred to a garden or a fairyland where she could never return again? But we can always return to our once-discovered fairyland. We can come as often as we want into our Dream Garden, our favorite place outdoors, which we are able to find anywhere we go or we can create our own—a place where we can restore and enjoy the magic of Nature, relax, rejuvenate, and live a healthy life filled with great books, beautiful flowers, mighty trees, and loving people.

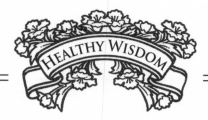

How far that little candle throws his beams!
So shines a good deed in a naughty world.

—*William Shakespeare (1564–1616), English playwright and poet*

Victory is the beautiful bright colored flower.

—*Sir Winston Churchill (1874–1965), British statesman, author, and prime minister*

The flowers that bloom in the spring bring to us a new life.

—*Unknown*

I know a bank whereon the wild thyme blows.

—*Shakespeare,* A Midsummer Night's Dream

There's rosemary, that's for remembrance;
and there is pansies, that's for thoughts.

—*Shakespeare,* Hamlet

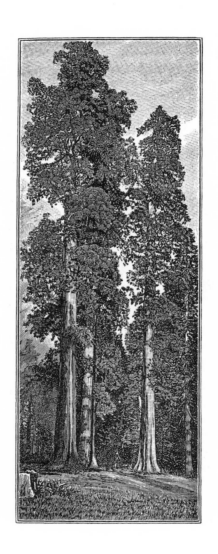

Chapter 12

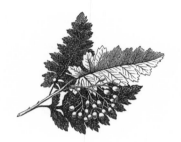

Dialogue with the Trees of Strength and Everlasting Life

Like a great poet, Nature is capable of producing the most stunning effects with the smallest means. Nature possesses only the sun, trees, flowers, water and love.

—*Henrich Heine (1797–1836), German poet and critic*

FACTS:

A forest is an ecosystem characterized by trees with a unique combination of plants, animals, microbes, soil, and climate. Twenty-seven percent of the world's total land area is covered in forests, which are home to more species of animals, birds, plants, and insects than any other environment on Earth. In the United States alone forests cover 747 million acres (301 million hectares) or 33 percent of the land base. Each year the forestry community plants 1½ billion tree seedlings in North America. This means more than six new trees for each North American. Satellite surveys confirm that across North America forests have actually expanded by 20 percent since 1970.

Forests are big factories producing oxygen. We need this product for our survival. Forests are greenhouse exchangers and clean our air by absorbing carbon dioxide and releasing oxygen. Trees lock in carbon dioxide and return it to the soil when they decompose instead of releasing it into the air and contributing to pollution. By taking in the amount of carbon we release into the atmosphere, trees help to reduce the "greenhouse" effect and remove the "carbon debt" we put into the environment. To grow a pound of wood, a tree uses 1.47 pounds of carbon dioxide and gives off 1.07 pounds of oxygen. One large growing tree can provide a day's oxygen for four people.[38] Perhaps no other activity involves so many people as outdoor recreation, which is a major land use of a quarter of a billion acres of public land and as much private land. More than 90 percent of the population participates. It is a $20 billion a year industry with an annual government investment of an additional $1 billion.[39]

The Druids, the wise priests of ancient Gaul, Celtic Britain, and Ireland, believed that trees transfer vital energy to us. The degree to which trees give us energy is determined by our birth date. Their religion focused on the worship of nature deities, and their rituals and ceremonies were held mostly in oak groves. The Druids believed that each of us has our own biological field and that everyone corresponds to a tree that is similar to the characteristics of his or her own bioenergetics. This particular tree is our talisman, a guardian of our health.

My talisman, predestined by Mother Nature, according to the Druids, is the cypress tree. I had been intuitively attracted to cypress trees all my life, and so I now understand why. It was one of the mysterious forces which world scientists will explain to all of us some day.

My cypress was special, good-looking, fresh, and slender. He was as tall as a pyramidal tower of a castle built many years ago by the grandest architect in the world—Mother Nature. His upper branches stretched like crooked arrows to the sky. I saw his outstanding beauty for the first time as I walked down a lane of these cone-bearing giants that stood like courageous guards forming a long green wall.

July was hot and steamy in Crimea when I returned again to this centuries-old park for a vacation. At noon I took refuge in the shade where trees cast their shadows on the forest path. I approached one of my special cypress trees, which stood proudly in line with so many others. His unusual dark green overlapping leaves formed a pattern against the sky that would have rivaled the most delicate Venetian lace.

I was happy to meet again with my old green friend. I tried to enfold him with my arms as much as I could to feel his intense energy. The tree's fragrant bark was slick with rainwater. "Salute, my friend! I have returned to see you again after a year," I whispered. He answered me with a shimmering rustle of his twisted, silky, smooth needles. I felt serene near this composed giant. An easy, relaxed mood and confidence returned to me as I received from this tree a new supply of vital energy along with a positive emotional state that had been nearly depleted by all the hard work I had done during the past year. Perhaps I was also influenced by my belief that I should begin every new year of my life here, near my cypress.

The first time I saw a cypress tree I couldn't understand why I was so attracted to it. I did not realize at the time that it had "called" me to it. Most people enjoy these evergreens as ornamental—a decoration; as an attribute to resorts; or as a material with which to build furniture, boats, or cedar chests. I admire cypress trees for another reason. I realize that pride and a strong spirit emanates from this tree. I believe that the dynamic intensity that propelled me to accomplish my dreams and goals came directly from this cypress.

Grandma used to say that trees and emerald green forests are the lungs and eyes of the earth, which supply us with the oxygen that we need to survive. "Trees are monuments to people who have died," she would say. "Nature gives these tree-monuments to those who are alive."

When I walk through a forest, I feel energized and rejuvenated. I never feel lonely around trees, the keepers of our life's secrets.

Every year our itinerary for summer vacation was the same. My first trip here was when I was three years old, and for many years thereafter just the four of us: Mama; Papa; my sister, Laura; and I enjoyed this beautiful resort. After our plane landed at Adler airport, we headed to picturesque Crimea. This prime destination was our favorite spot—a place where friendly cypresses and oleanders swayed in the fresh breeze from the clear turquoise sea and a profusion of golden orange magnolia blooms greeted its visitors. It seems that when people immerse themselves in this special Mediterranean microclimate, they are rejuvenated.

Our cab driver sped along the twisting road through the mountains. The road was difficult and we were nervous, but he seemed to be an attentive driver. One side of the mountains held an open view of the sea. The road, bathed in bright sunshine, was perched high in the air. Beams of light stretched from the sun to the sea where they scattered over the sea's surface like sugar crystals on a frosted cake. All year I had waited to visit this salubrious place that seemed to pulse with vibrant, vital energy.

This year our parents had promised us a big surprise and I was anxious to see it. After several minutes Mama asked our driver to stop and we stepped out of the car.

"Look at the tops of the mountains," Mama said.

The profile of a woman's face, formed by the mountains and resembling the Russian Empress, Catherine the Great, was immortalized in stone by the most amazing sculptor in the world—Mother Nature. It was a striking and welcoming gate to our beautiful destination—Crimea.

Crimea is a peninsula between the Black Sea and the Sea of Azov. Its climate is similar to that of northern California with its cool and breezy mornings and evenings. Its copious mountains, tall trees, and subtropical exotic plants created a lavish panorama, and its warm azure seawater was luxurious to bathe in.

The northern side of Crimea is a steppe, covered with rich wild grasses and field flowers. The Crimean Mountains stand on the southern side.

Crimea is known for its more than 600 curative and preventive health centers, many curative mud deposits, 200 mineral springs, and essential oils.

Yalta, the largest city in Crimea, is home to a famous health resort that opened in 1783. Its inhabitants pass on ancient legends of this city's origins from generation to generation.

In ancient times ships were sent out to discover foreign shores from the capital of the Byzantine Empire, Constantinople. The voyage was not easy. The explorers met violent storms on the Black Sea. A thick fog rested on the waves and often obscured the horizon. For many days the explorers drifted aimlessly. When water and food supplies dwindled on the ships, the exhausted sailors lost their will to go on and simply waited to die.

One morning a light, saving breeze began to blow and slowly dissipated the milky shroud of fog. In the bright sunlight the explorers saw green and purple mountains in the distance. Their journey would become easier now that the fog had lifted.

"Yalos! Yalos!" A sailor on watch cried out the Greek word for shore.

They had found the wonderful Tavrida (Crimea), where there was no snowy winter and the fresh, healing air held the scent of the sea and the aroma of herbs. The low spirits of the tired explorers were lifted. They manned their oars and directed their ship toward the calling shore. On the fertile land, among the natives, they founded a small colony and named it Yalos. From then on, the city was called Yalta.

Yalta is the main city in Crimea, with a population of about 85,000. The Russian author Anton Chekhov wrote his best novels and stage plays there, and Russian tsars and their families vacationed each July at the beautiful palace in Livadia, several miles north of Yalta.

Every morning of our vacation in Yalta, we opened the big Venetian windows in our spacious apartment on the beach and gazed at the endless expanse of sea and sunny, blue sky. Before going to sleep at night, we were again attracted by the sky, this time to gaze at the Milky Way, which looked like millions of stars had been swept across the sky in a single brush stroke. There in Crimea I saw closely for the first time stars falling toward earth and never reaching it. They burned up so fast.

"Look, a star fell!" exclaimed Laura.

"They say that when a star falls, a person dies. A star cannot live when there is no energy to keep it burning. It's the same for people," I told her.

"This is very sad, but it is so beautiful at the same time," continued my sister.

"As a child, I dreamed of igniting the stars. It seemed that if you could keep them illuminated, no one would die. And my magical stars would not fall so suddenly and quickly out of the sky," said Mama softly.

With the midnight blue sky as a backdrop the lighthouse clearly stood out, but the stars shone above it like fireflies in a woodland village of fairies. Suddenly a second star fell and cascaded through the sky.

"Oh, my God! It's really scary," I said.

"Don't be afraid of falling stars," responded Papa. "Better make a wish quickly. I know your wish will come true if you want something good to happen."

We closed our eyes and made a wish to return to Crimea next summer, where we could easily breathe in the fresh fragrance of cypresses and listen to the sound of sea waves with foam-white crests rolling to the shore.

"You know, girls, it is true that some stars quietly witness death, but I never was afraid when I saw them," said Mama. "A white falling star is the shadow of a person who has passed away; it is his echo. Everyone has his own star. It lives in the sky while the person walks the earth. But there are silver falling stars, which bring hope and grant wishes. You can easily recognize the silver ones. They are usually bigger and brighter when they descend from the sky."

"Girls, come close. I will tell you a fairy tale about how children threw the sun into the sky. My grandma told me this when I was a little boy," Papa said.

A long time ago the sun was a human who had two bright lights under his arms. When he raised his hand, the earth was illuminated with sun-beams, as it is now with electricity. When he went to bed, everything plunged into cold and darkness. People didn't want to live in darkness and decided that children must fetch the Sun Man and take him to the sky.

This decision was passed down from generation to generation. One day some children sneaked up on the Sun Man when he was sleeping. They took him by force and threw him like a ball to the sky. Those children had forgotten that their elders had told them to treat the Sun gently. Since then the Sun walks on the sky, lighting up everything around. When the Sun rises, he sends away the cold and darkness and his light spills all over the earth and warms every living thing: people, trees, plants, flowers, and animals.

But at night the Moon came to the sky. Nobody expected that the Sun would see the Moon at this time. When the Sun saw the Moon, he pierced her through with one of his sharp knife-like beams. The Moon was badly hurt and begged the Sun for mercy. She asked the powerful Sun if she could at least keep her backbone. The Sun was a generous person and allowed the Moon to keep her backbone. She was still sick when she returned home and remained hidden for several days, but soon the Moon recovered from her wounds and appeared again in the sky. Each day she grew larger and larger until she became whole and full. And that happens every time the Moon enters the sky.

"That is the end of my story," said Papa.

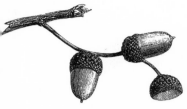We listened to the sound of waves crested in white foam rolling slowly to the shore. As if on cue, the midnight-blue sea suddenly became antique gold in the middle as the full moon blazed her path through the sea.

"It is known that at such times of full moonlight great writers were inspired to create their best romantic poems," added Papa. "Tomorrow will probably be a beautiful, romantic day."

The next morning the gentle sound of the blue sea woke me up. It always seemed as if it beckoned to me to come and swim in its grandeur. I enjoyed a refreshing swim every morning at sunrise and then carried renewed energy throughout the day ahead. I felt ready to absorb new and exciting impressions from the beautiful surroundings.

Clusters of oleander rustled their narrow green leaves, and pink cyclamen flowers basked in the sun, raising their heads to the sky as Yalta awakened slowly and lazily. Under the rising sun vacationers began to fill the soft, golden sand beaches. But we had already enjoyed the water and were ready to explore new areas of Crimea.

Often Mama and Papa would entertain my sister and me after the beach with promenades in the magnificent Crimean Mountain Forest Preserve. There we had unforgettable journeys in oak, pine, and beech forests surrounded by mountains. This huge park was founded in 1923 as the Crimean Hunting Preserve. There people hunted and enjoyed the thick forests in a climate that healed body and soul.

On the northwestern side of the Crimean peninsula were the Swan's Islands, where we walked through alpine meadows and emerald groves of pines, oaks, and hornbeams. Giant pines stood in all their mighty power and noble beauty. Their ruddy trunks and deep green needles towered above the other trees. They appeared to be close, but at the same time far away, wrapped up around the Crimean Mountains. Rocking gently under a warm breeze from the Black Sea, they witnessed through many sunny springs and summers the dreams and hopes of all the different people who visited the park.

The energy of the pine tree, according to the Druid's horoscope, corresponds to people who are born from February 19-28 and from August 24-September 2. The Latin name for pine is *Pinus*, which means a rock, and like a rock, the pine is strong with a firm trunk and roots and does not demand any special treatment. The same can be said for "pine people."

My youngest son, Yuri, was born on August 29. Now he is 24 years old. He is a young "pine" man. When he was a baby, I would give him baths infused with pine needles. Pine baths invigorate the body and can be a blessing when we are overtired at the end of a workday. It can be especially beneficial to people who work in the sports and fitness fields.

Bathing in fragrant aromatic pine water can make you feel alert, cheerful, and refreshed while restoring your energy. The aroma of pine comes from its essential oils, which act as a pain reliever, a disinfectant, and an anti-inflammatory agent. They stimulate the immune system and improve the metabolism.

If you are overtired, suffer from a headache, or want to improve your mood, try a pine bath:

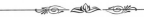

1. Fill the bathtub with warm water and dissolve in it 3½ ounces of liquid pine concentrate or two ounces of pine powder. You can also use an infusion of pine needles. Take a warm, but not hot, pine bath for 10–15 minutes.

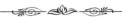

A pine bath is beneficial to us because the essential oils of this tree evaporate easily and fill the air with the smallest high-energy particles carrying an electric charge. When we breathe in ionized air, it greatly heals our body and it acts as a calming, natural remedy. This is important to know because many of us don't realize that we are always undergoing a so-called green phytoncide starvation because we live far away from the forests. Only on occasion do we take a walk in a forest. People who live close to forests are more often able to walk in them. It is unfortunate that many of us rarely have the opportunity and pleasure to communicate with pines, our green giants.

Grandma kept on the window sill an opened, small glass bottle with essential oils of pine, linden, birch, lavender, or peppermint. It increased the biological activity of the air in our house and it made positive changes in our health. It helped to propel the hidden reserves of our bodies toward well-being. I try to live the way that Grandma did, and so bottles of these essential oils are a permanent fixture in my house.

One summer my husband, Greg, Yuri, and I went to Pitsunda, a small town on the shore of the Black Sea at the foot of a steep mountain in the high Caucasian Mountains. He was three years old and it was the first trip of his life. We enjoyed the month we spent there. It was a month filled with swimming and breathing fresh air or "heliotherapy," as we like to call it. We relaxed on sandy beaches, bordered by huge boulders that resembled knights from a fairy tale. We took trips and walked in the shadowy grove of ancient pines in Pitsunda, which supplied shipbuilders for many centuries with the strongest wood.

This small town on the cape was founded by the ancient Greeks as a Middle Age city together with Port Piteous, in Greek *Pityus*. It still maintains parts of its ancient fort walls, which house the Byzantine era basilica, a cathedral built in the tenth century. We made the trip again and again through this ancient, sacred place that keeps the secrets and myths of one of the small parts of Europe from the Middle Ages.

We walked with Yuri every day underneath a canopy of lofty branches in this centuries-old pine grove. It was warm, cozy, and quiet. Yuri walked slowly, his tiny feet treading carefully on dried pine needles that formed a thick cushion on the ground. "Mama, I want to live here forever!" Yuri said.

This had been his first meeting with a tree-friend that was predetermined by Nature on the day he was born. Yuri wanted to visit the pine grove everyday. As a small boy, he couldn't explain *why* he wanted to go to the pines, but a connection already had been made.

The following year we went to Yaremcha, a small town in the Carpathian Mountains. On a sunny winter day we took our skis into a forest that shone with radiant downy snow and smelled deliciously of powerful pines and beeches. Fresh air flowed into our lungs and filled us with joy. The forest was quiet. The snow looked like beautiful lace tatting of diamond stars and sunbeams. The trees were dressed in the snow's bright, white diaphanous coat, and the silver-green pines had faded into the milky atmosphere.

"Are we in a fairy tale kingdom, Mama?" my son asked me.

"Yes, we are," I whispered. "Do you remember when I read you a poem written by Alexander Pushkin about the forest in winter and your favorite pines?"

"Yes, I remember," Yuri said with great inspiration. "I'll begin, but you continue, because I am not sure I know all of it." He turned towards the pines and began:

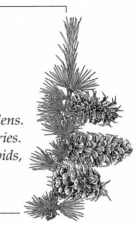

There is a forest in front of us.
I remember the pines
And their divine beauty.
All of their branches are hidden
By the sheds of snow to the tops
Of the asps, birches and naked lindens.
It shines a ray of the night luminaries.
There is no road; the shrubs, the rapids,
All snow-bound by a snow storm,
Deeply in the snow tucked in.

We spent three hours in the forest on the mountain. Afterwards we rushed off to the Russian steaming *banya* (sauna). The banya was built of logs that absorbed the fragrances of various aromatic and resinous matters and phytoncides. We could chose from among besoms of oak, linden, birch, eucalyptus, silver fir, nettle, and pine. The besoms clean the air in the banya and act as an antibacterial agent, helping our skin and lungs stay healthy. The fresh fragrance of a forest permeated this woody steaming chamber when we used silver fir besom, rich in resins, essential oil, phytoncides, and vitamin C. The aroma of pine or silver fir needles in a besom for the sauna contain bactericidal phytoncides. It is considered to be an excellent remedy for treating lethargy, catarrh, bronchitis, laryngitis, and pharyngytis. After steaming with pine besoms, our skin had a sweet, fresh smell and a healthy glow for a long time.

Essential oils act as a bactericidal on the skin. If you take a smear from any external part of your body for microscopic examination after steaming with these besoms, you will not find even one microbe on your skin. We felt refreshed and had tons of energy. The explanation is simple: This method of cleaning opened the pores of our skin, and toxins were expelled. Toxins are hidden enemies and poison the blood. When we remove them on a regular basis, we can keep ourselves well. After you steam in a sauna, it is beneficial to drink one of the following four vitamin teas:

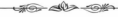

2. Mix one tablespoon each of rose hips berries and black currants.

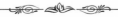

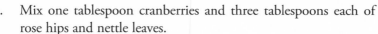

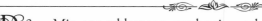 3. Mix one tablespoon cranberries and three tablespoons each of rose hips and nettle leaves.

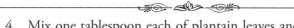

4. Mix one tablespoon each of plantain leaves and mountain ash berries.

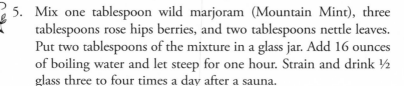

5. Mix one tablespoon wild marjoram (Mountain Mint), three tablespoons rose hips berries, and two tablespoons nettle leaves. Put two tablespoons of the mixture in a glass jar. Add 16 ounces of boiling water and let steep for one hour. Strain and drink ½ glass three to four times a day after a sauna.

We took two branches of a one-year-old pine back to our hotel room. One branch we put in a vase with water to refresh the air. The second, we used to make a special vitamin drink.

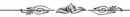

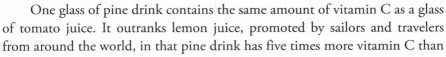 6. Preparation of this drink is simple and quick, but only the needles of a one-year-old pine should be used. Wash two ounces of pine needles and grind them in a porcelain mortar. Then add two to three glasses of boiling water and let steep in a cool, dark place for two hours. Add honey and lemon, according to taste. Strain and drink immediately. If the drink is stored, it will lose vitamins.

One glass of pine drink contains the same amount of vitamin C as a glass of tomato juice. It outranks lemon juice, promoted by sailors and travelers from around the world, in that pine drink has five times more vitamin C than lemon juice.

The branches of the trees in the forest played a nice melody as they swished under the light wind of a frosty winter night. My little son was in bed and I told him a story about my pine.

I was 10 years old, and for the first time in my life, I had climbed up to the top of the pine growing near our house. I imagined that I was atop the mast of a flagship. The wind was shaking the tree. My pine vessel was rocking in unison with all other trees around. The rustle of the leaves resembled the sound of broiling ocean waves before a storm. From atop the tree I saw how the forest opened its boundless space to many other green trees. The spacious green distance, gold light and shadow, and a caressing play of the brightest greens and sunbeams mixed with the solemn tranquility of Nature.

I knocked three times on the trunk of the pine. "Do you hear me, my friend? Please take away forever any illnesses and misfortunes from my family!"

My grandma believed that if you knock on a tree, no one can bewitch you with the "evil eye." She was sure that if you pass a tree and touch a branch of it, any harmful aspects of your life are sifted through the tree's chlorophyll and the tree then gives off a fresh flow of energy that transforms any negative energy affecting your life into positive energy.

One day when I was a child, our next-door neighbor came to our house to consult with Mama. While she was waiting, she spoke with me about my crafts. Suddenly Grandma came into the house and right away took this woman from me, asking how she could help her. When our neighbor left, Grandma said, "Go outside and knock on the tree!"

"What's the matter?" I asked.

"This lady has 'bad eyes,'" Grandma answered. "Do you understand me?"

I went outside to our pine and knocked on it three times. My grandma trusted in the power of thought. She believed that if you feel that you can do something to prevent harmful things in your life from happening; you just might be able to do it.

Grandma felt closely tied to the trees, and the same day she explained to me what she meant when she said the woman had "bad" eyes. She felt that some people are born with the ability to bewitch others by looking at them and thereby passing on to them negative, destructive energy, which at some time could adversely affect their life. She believed passionately that trees can save us from it and she could tell many stories to prove her theory.

I began to observe people's eyes in a different way. I look at the expression in their eyes. Are they cool or warm, kind or wild, caressing or loving, romantic, thoughtful, smart, or foggy? Are these eyes strong, powerful, or quickly running from one subject to another, like checking everybody and everything? Are they slow moving and pensive?

"People's eyes are the mirror of their soul," Grandma liked to say. She was absolutely right. I have noticed that when people are happy, their eyes shine.

If they are unhappy, their eyes have no light within. I adopted Grandma's practice of knocking on a tree to drive away the evil eye. And again and again I have noticed that trees seem to come to the rescue. When I asked Grandma when she started to believe that trees could rid us of troubles, she told me that she had read about this centuries-old tradition in old books, inherited from *her* grandma. She trusted this simple human wisdom and experienced the healing energy from trees that she touched in her own life. She became confident that it worked for her.

Grandma told me that in ancient times soldiers would search for a tree to touch to draw from its energy source for faster recovery from battle wounds. The Druids, the wise priests of the forests in Great Britain, were some of the first to believe this. Pine and oak were considered the most effective in "green therapy." Ancient soldiers tried to "drink" a tree's energy before they took part in fighting on the battlefields of bloody wars. Trees helped them because they are sacred creatures—Nature's messengers.

I was so inspired by the soldiers' story that I painted a picture in watercolors of how I believed that scene might have looked. I never was a great artist, but Grandma loved it and hung in our house. She was proud that teaching me about the world of Nature often brought positive results. I tried to show her how grateful I was.

Grandma often talked to her plants. She told me she always knew what kind of mood they were in. I watched her sometimes. She would speak to her plants as if they were human.

"Why do you speak with flowers, Grandma?" I asked her one day. I was careful not to be unkind to her. I didn't want to say, "Hey, Grandma, that looks and sounds crazy!"

Grandma answered, "It is difficult to explain, but I tamed (domesticated) them and they always remind me to be cheerful."

Then Grandma broke into a story, which she called "Three Daughters, Three Trees."

A fisherman lived with his wife on the sea-shore, nine miles from the small town of Alushta in Crimea," Grandma began. "They were kind, honest, and hard-working people and always ready to give shelter to occasional travelers and share their last piece of bread with people less fortunate.

"It is said that the locals highly respected the fisherman and his wife. But the people's good opinions were countered by the bad opinions of the couple harbored by their own children, their three daughters.

"The oldest daughter, Poplar, was unattractive, short and clumsy, and hostile in nature. To disparage her parents, she would listen in on their private conversations and repeat what they had said to everyone in the seaside village.

"The second daughter, Pomegranate, was obsessed with the color pink. She criticized her parents because she was not beautiful with rosy cheeks. She imagined that if she became a rose, passersby would stop and look at her with admiration.

"The youngest daughter, Cypress, was beautiful and possessed a merry personality. But under the influence of her older sisters she also thought negatively about her father and mother. She was unhappy that her parents gave birth to her at night instead of day, which explained why she was so quick and easily amused.

"It was hard for the parents to be ridiculed by their children, but what could be done? Their love was blind and helpless. They tolerated their children's taunts and rude behavior. To avoid attention, they often traveled to the mountains and lived there for days at a time.

"One day while the parents were at home, all three daughters, angered by an event outside, broke into the cabin and attacked their mother and father.

"'Oh, skies!' the parents prayed. 'Is there any power that can defend us from our children?'

"Before they could finish their prayers, a voice sounded, 'Poplar! You forsake your parents because you are a dwarf, so become a towering tree with no fruits or flowers. Not one bird, except the crow, will nest in you.'

"'Pomegranate! Your wish will also come true. You'll become a tree with pink flowers, and everyone will stop and look at them in admiration, but no one will lean over to smell these beautiful flowers because they won't have a scent. Your fruits, bright red in the middle, will not satiate anyone's hunger or quench anyone's thirst because they will not ripen.'

"'Cypress! The fate of your sisters will also be yours. You complained about your merry personality. You will become a beautiful but sad tree.'

"Startled, the girls fled from the cabin. Their parents ran after them, but their children were nowhere to be seen. Three mysterious trees stood in the yard. One raised its branches high as if it wanted to become taller. The second was covered with pink flowers. The third was frozen in sad silence.

"The trees were then named after the three daughters, Poplar, Pomegranate, and Cypress."

"You see," said Grandma, "three daughters of a fisherman, Poplar, Pomegranate, and Cypress, demanded too much from their parents and treated them badly until they got what they wished for. Trees are like people."

Grandma shared with me an interesting old book on natural healing that described a rowan tree. This tree has plenty of unusual features. The rowan tree is said to bring luck and happiness to a house. I have seen how young rowans were planted near houses in the Baltic states of Lithuania, Latvia, and Estonia in Karelia (northwestern Russia). In Russia there are 34 kinds of fruit and decorative trees. Rowan or Mountain Cranberry tree contains sugar, organic acids, vitamins A and C, and tanning matters.

People planted these trees near their windows and believed that no wicked person would dare pass the threshold of their house. People believed and created a lovely ritual of placing a branch of rowan tree in the shoes of a future bride and groom before their marriage ceremony to wish them happiness from the bottom of the heart and to prevent any misfortune in their future life "for better or worse."

The national emblems of some countries feature images of flowers or leaves. Such countries as France, Canada, Haiti, Cyprus, and Lebanon use the lily, a maple leaf, palm, or olive branch.

I have seen photographs of famous yoga instructors sitting under a sacred tree. Yoga schools identify human beings with trees and the human body with a temple.[40] A trunk of a tree is a brain; the branches are 72,000 nerves; seven flowers on a tree are seven centers of the astral body; the leaves are lungs. This is not only an analogy or a supposition, but scientists in Russia have discovered that trees vibrate and have negative or positive moods and operate with a nervous system much like that of a human.

I think Grandma was right about a lot of things. She had such a close connection to Nature and she loved her daily gardening. Sometimes she helped Grandpa care for the vineyard. Plants and trees became for her a source of education about our life, which comes from Nature, and she learned how to lead a natural life and stay away from all the toxins, chemicals, and poisons that destroy our health. She taught us with her uncompromising commitment to everything natural, clean, and healthy.

I remember a quiet afternoon in the forest near our summerhouse when I was small. The birds were twittering. A dried twig crunched under my foot and interrupted the silence of the forest and the life of its inhabitants. A narrow path led me to a clearing that was bathed in sunlight. I stopped there and listened and noticed that the forest's silence wasn't really silent. There was an active life going on within it, indeed. The trees worked hard, bringing out phytoncides and specific fermentation to help people, birds, animals, insects, and themselves.

I found myself near an aspen. Grandma revered this powerful tree. I saw how she had listened to the tremble or "quake" of the aspen leaves. She said that when the aspen quakes, it is driving away "evil spirits" and keeping people from diseases.

The apple and laurel, on the other hand, in ancient times were called "lightning conductors" and could divert lightning if they were planted near houses. This happens because of the trees' miraculous ability to energize fields around them. Plants polarize the air and create electrical charges by exuding essential oils, which influence the formation of thunderstorms and lightning.

Plants are our sponsors and amulets on the thorny path of our lives. In the golden times, it is said, verbena gave people love and a joyful mood; elder was a symbol of diligence; buckthorn protected people from witchcraft; the leaves of a fig tree were used for fortune-telling and its branches saved matadors from angry bulls.

The black mulberry tree is said to support success in business and is ruled by the planet Mercury, a sponsor of entrepreneurial people. It is believed that the ash tree brings happiness to the home. Aloe gives prosperity and long life to the people who keep this plant in their houses. It is easy to explain why. Aloe can live and blossom without water for several years. The tradition to hang aloe on doors or windows was popular in ancient Egypt. Cyclamen is well known as the plant amulet and a guardian from all troubles. This belief came from ancient Rome. From Hippocrates' time, cyclamen was said to heal nervous diseases, stomach and intestinal disorders, colds, and rheumatism.

I remember how Grandma invented her own natural treatments for sleeplessness and headaches. The simplest remedy was to keep pots of geraniums on the window sills. The secret was that geranium plants absorb all harmful substances and microbes from the air—even humidity and smoke. Scientists in Europe confirmed that phytoncides of this flower efficiently remove microbes and its aroma promotes sound sleep.

There is little doubt that plants and trees greatly influence our lives. All day long the forest sounds like a symphonic orchestra with mysterious signals sent by plants and trees to each other. Scientists continue their experiments to determine what these signals mean.

The Russian scientist, Victor F. Vostokov, a world-known specialist of Tibetan medicine, believes that we can feel how "prana" or living energy flows from the top of a tree. I experienced the energy flow from a tree for the first time in a forest when I noticed that one tree stood out from the rest. Intuitively I put my arms around the tree and hugged it with all my heart. I felt its vibrant, warm biological field. I closed my eyes and envisioned its roots and the earth's juices moving to the roots from underground. These vital juices of life had been flowing inside of its trunk to the top of its crown. I heard its rapid and unceasing run. It was early spring, when the motion of Nature's juices can be heard clearly if one stops to listen. I felt the living energy fill the tree.

It is the same with us, if we identify ourselves with a tree. We will experience in ourselves the movement of ascending and descending energy. In this way we can "flush out" our neuroses and cope with life's pressure. Many people, after communicating with a tree, feel at peace.

After having my first and unforgettable *tête-à-tête* with this maple, I stroked his trunk with my hand as if it were a growing child. I touched its silky, tri-pointed, and thin-veined leaves. They were trembling and passing on their joy of life to me.

When we feel upset or unhappy, experience a loss of energy, or are struggling with problems or disease in our lives, we must not forget to turn to our friends, the trees, for help. They are always ready to answer our call and infuse us with their revitalizing energy.

American poet Robert Frost expressed his love for Nature and trees in "The Sound of Trees" and "Tree at My Window" with his lyrical language, as did naturalists Henry David Thoreau and John Muir.

Thoreau wrote in his first book a passage called "Autumn":

> *As we lay awake long before daybreak, listening to the rippling of the river and the rustling of the leaves, in suspense whether the wind blew up or down the stream, was favorable or unfavorable to our voyage, we already suspected that there was a change in the weather, from a freshness as of autumn in these sounds. The wind in the woods sounded like an incessant waterfall dashing and roaring amid rocks, and we even felt encouraged by the unusual activity of the elements. He who hears the rippling of rivers in these degenerate days will not utterly despair. That night was the turning point in the season. We had gone to bed in summer, and awoke in autumn, for summer passes into autumn in some unimaginable point of time, like the turning of a leaf.[41]*

As a naturalist, explorer, and writer, Muir left us an enduring legacy. He founded the well-known Sierra Club while lobbying as an activist and a writer for the establishment of Yosemite National Park. John Muir shares with us his observations and some of the wonders he found in the great forests of the West.

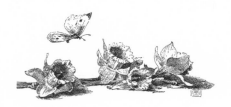

We all travel the Milky Way together; trees and men; but it never occurred to me until this stormy day, while swinging in the wind, that trees are travelers, in the ordinary sense. They make many journeys, not extensive ones, it is true; but our own little journeys, away and back again, are only little more than tree-wavings—many of them not so much.

When the storm began to abate, I dismounted and sauntered down through the calming woods. The storm-tones died away, and, turning toward the cast, I beheld the countless hosts of the forest hushed and tranquil, towering above one another on the slopes of the hills like a devout audience. The setting sun filled them with amber light, and seemed to say, while they listened, "My peace I give unto you."[42]

In addition to Frost, Thoreau, and Muir, many others have penned their reverence for nature. In 1913, poet Joyce Kilmer graciously wrote of his love and admiration for powerful creations of nature in his beautiful poem *Trees*. He compared a tree with a poem and described that a tree "looks at God all day and lifts her leafy arms to pray". I wonder, if it is a coincidence between this poem and a story in prose once told to me by Marion, a good and wise friend and neighbor? Marion is 84 years old. She is still a very beautiful, statuesque lady and carries herself with great dignity. I call her "My Victorian Lady." You will not meet this special breed very often today.

When Marion was born in 1923 on a picturesque farm in Pennsylvania, her parents planted a small sugar maple near their farm house to celebrate her birth. So, Marion and Sugar, her tree-friend, grew up together. Marion played near her maple. She liked to stroke the smooth grey-brown bark that covered the trunk. She often hugged her tree and shared secret thoughts with it.

One day, while Marion watched her mother tap the sap from the sugar maple and make her delicious maple syrup, she thought it must be painful for the tree to give all she had—her vital juices. She felt so sorry for her friend. She hugged her tree with all her heart and asked her how she was feeling and what she could do for her. The sun shone through the bright green leaves at the top of the tree. Pale green leaves below shimmered with a satin finish sparkle reminiscent of invisible silver stars in the sky that sometimes can be seen in the daylight. The sugar maple stood like a pretty young woman, lifting her strong leafy arms to the sky. Her leaves trembled slightly in unison with the wind. Then Marion heard a quiet, tender murmur. Her tree-friend was sending back to her all she had to give, her positive energy and strength.

My good friend, Jan Marie Werblin Kemp, recalls how childhood visits to her grandmother's country home fostered in her a profound love of Nature and especially trees.

> *I climbed the steep quartz gravel drive to my grandmother's house, past clumps of the tiniest purple forget-me-nots, smatterings of bright yellow daffodils, mammoth stalks of purple velvet hollyhocks, white "snowball" bushes, pink peonies, ice-blue hydrangea. The air in spring was alive with the buzzing of honeybees, fluttering butterflies and hummingbirds.*
>
> *And, in a clearing, atop the hill, barely visible from the winding road that cut through Maryland's rural pastures in the 1950s, sat my grandmother's brown-shingled house nestled in a sylvan setting—sky-high poplars, red maples, blue spruces, mighty oaks and chestnut trees.*
>
> *I often heard them speak as they bent under the weight of the wind. Acorns crunched under my feet as I walked beneath the oaks, and a blanket of soft fragrant needles beckoned me to lie down and rest beneath a blue spruce that swept the clouds away with its feathery branches.*
>
> *Deeper in the woods, where the air is heady and rich with oxygen, a fallen log lay rotting on parched brown leaves. A microcosm of life had made that log its world. Lichens crowned the crumbling bark; worms wound their way in and out of round holes. And from the disintegration, new tree shoots pushed out from the rich brown humus the dead tree had become. As I studied that log, I realized that I was learning an immensely valuable life lesson. Within the serenity of the forest, alone with the log, I learned that living organisms never die, they merely change their form. Trees, like humans, are sacrosanct and eternal.*

Mother Nature built a bridge of communion between plants and us on our birthdays. Come to your tree. Snuggle up to it and listen carefully to the quiet rustle of its leaves. Bond with your tree and it will share its magic with you. If you have even a small piece of land near your home, plant your own tree and enjoy its energy.

As a child I thought that all artists were humans, but I was wrong and I'll tell you why. I drew primitive pictures of flowers and trees and unusual plants. When I became a journalist and traveled a lot, I always carried with me an album and crayons. New drawings appeared in my sketchbook: old buildings in various cities, people's faces, scenery. These sketches always reminded me of visits to unknown places and meetings with interesting people. When I drew Nature scenes, I discovered fresh beauty in each new picture. In my sketchbook appeared trees covered with a young, delicate green coat in spring's forest and bright, sometimes fluorescent flowers and golden wheat ripening in the fields in summer. In autumn my album held pictures of rust-colored blooming wild flowers and countless red-yellow-orange-green leaves, falling everywhere and celebrating the last days of their lives.

One day I realized who the true artists were. I understood that the most talented artists on earth are not people, but all the seasons of the year: winter, spring, summer, and fall. We human beings just duplicate what Mother Nature created.

On the first day of fall some years ago, this autumn-artist had used already all of her unique palette of colors: green and yellow, gold, orange, and burgundy. I came to the small pictorial village in Moldova, in the southeastern part of Europe, on assignment from a newspaper for young readers. This village was well known, thanks to an old gigantic oak tree that lived high upon a hill.

On the world map this small country looks curiously like a bunch of grapes and is situated on the major European crossroads. For many centuries Moldova attracted numerous invaders: Scythians, Hottentots, Huns, Golden Horde of Tatars, and Mongolians. From the twelfth century this grape country was a part of the Great Roman, Ottoman, Russian tsar's, and Soviet empires, and Romania.

I stood near the Herculean oak on a hill. In the heat of the summer he covered the village and its inhabitants in shaded coolness, taking them under his wide and branching crown. Even travelers passing by would stop near the old oak to rest. In the fall the land near the oak was covered with a blanket of his lacy, colored patterned leaves. In the winter the oak stood and met with great joy the rare and timid sunbeams which sometimes appeared in the heavy, gray sky.

Fall came to the village with September and the first toll of the school bell. The day was warm, dry, and sunny, and after lessons a group of seventh graders took a walk in the forest that was bedecked in full crimson-gold attire.

Autumn, the great artist that she is, generously spent all her rich and beautiful colors to adorn the trees. She covered maples and lindens with gold brocade. The birches she painted with ochre, but the leaves of the aspens she rouged with red. Pine and fir trees were renewed with rich dark-green color.

Autumn swept the fields and meadows and left them standing in a burnt sienna, waiting for winter. She gathered sweet-scented bales of hay in the meadows and stacked them like the towers of an ancient castle.

Fall took good care of the Herculean oak standing alone on the hill for more than 200 years. She dressed the giant tree in copper-forged armor, and he looked like a king's knight.

Andrew, one of the seventh graders, walked together with his classmates in the forest, and they came across the oak. The tree allowed a light breeze to ruffle slowly the smaller branches along its strong arms.

"Oak branches are so strong," Andrew thought. "I can make a good stick from one." He bent one of the branches and a crackle sounded so sorrowfully that the astonished boy stopped. Immediately another boy's voice rang out, "All come here! Look at this daredevil!" Boys and girls came running to the outcry of the red-headed boy. They cried with indignation, "Did you plant this tree? Who gave you the right to hurt our favorite oak?"

Andrew realized that his schoolmates were not joking with him and that they were not going to forgive him the damage he had done to the tree. He began to run to save himself from being beaten by the children, but the children caught him and under their tough escort he was taken to a house. Their knock on the door brought outside a tall, gray-haired man dressed in a business suit. It appeared as if he was dressed for an important meeting. His jacket was adorned with many medals honoring his achievements in World War II. When the boy saw them, he became ashamed of what he did. He began to mumble, trying to justify himself, "I just wanted to make a stick for our game *gorodky* or I thought I could make a tool to shoot the crows."

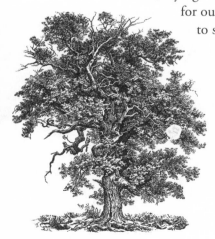

"Don't listen to him, Uncle Basil!" the boys and girls said. "He is a real forest's hooligan."

Uncle Basil turned to Andrew and asked in a quiet voice, "Well, what do you think, boy? Are you a hooligan? I cannot believe that you could be so cruel to a tree, especially our oak." He continued, "Unfortunately I don't have time now to discuss this, but please come tomorrow to our club."

He addressed the other students, "You, boys and girls, come on time. Don't be late."

"Uncle Basil, we'll go with you to the village hall," said the students and they did. It looked as if they had forgotten all about Andrew. He trailed them slowly. They stopped near the village hall where Uncle Basil was. Andrew looked around while the group made final plans to meet tomorrow at the club. Near the road, not far away he noticed two rowan trees, trampled down. These young trees, glistening with red berries, were broken in half. Andrew realized that they would not grow anymore—they would not produce oxygen or delight people's eyes.

Andrew approached Uncle Basil and silently showed him what had happened to the rowan trees. Uncle Basil shrugged his shoulders and said sadly, "During World War II when our Army passed through the territory of fascist Germany, we didn't crush with our tanks and military cars any of the trees and other foliage. We passed near them, but we did everything possible to keep them safe from harm. In spite of that, it was Germany and Hitler, the land of our enemies. But now, in peaceful times, we have here some people who don't want to preserve Nature in their Motherland."

Andrew dropped his eyes and said, "I will plant two or three new rowan trees. Please let me make it up to you and correct my mistake with the oak."

The red-headed boy, who first caught Andrew near the oak, said, "You will plant. Sure, you will plant. But we will not accept you as a member of our club, 'Good Friends of the Forest.' I don't think so."

Andrew was shocked. All he wanted most now was to become a member of their friendly green team. So Andrew said goodbye and went home. The next day he went to the park after school. He became more and more interested in Nature. Suddenly in a beautiful meadow in the park he saw a small, agile girl. She was standing near a goat, which was nibbling fresh grass. Andrew began to cry loudly with indignation, "Ah, you, the hooligan! What are you doing?"

He rushed up to the girl and said, "Immediately go out and find another, more appropriate place for your goat!" The girl didn't expect anybody to see what she was allowing her goat to do and so she became frightened. She pulled the goat's horns, but the stubborn animal refused to stop and continued to nibble the grass on the park's lawn.

Then Andrew lost his patience. He came up behind the goat and clapped his hands loudly. The goat turned and ran full speed through the park. The girl ran away after her. Andrew followed them, running so fast that he caught them both. He took the goat's horn, then the girl's arm and escorted them to the club, "Good Friends of the Forest." So Andrew became a faithful guard of green verdure. Members of the club accepted him and recognized that he did very well with the goat and the girl.

He asked Uncle Basil why the boys became so angry with him in the forest near the oak. Even then he was thinking that no harm would be done if you break just one branch of an old big oak because the tree is strong and can survive some damage. The boys and girls heard his questions to Uncle Basil. One of them said passionately, "You know what? You know nothing; you are a fool if you think that. This oak that you hurt is a famous, historical tree."

Uncle Basil asked Andrew, "Do you not know what this oak is all about?"

Andrew had no idea. "OK," said Uncle Basil. "We'll explore the oak's history in the forest." And they went to the hill where the ancient oak was standing as a guard and a wonderful monument to Mother Nature. Over the years it had become an inseparable part of the village's history. It stands today because in their turn the village people carefully guarded their most famous inhabitant. Over the years many storms swept over the oak, but it remained standing. The old oak was named Suvorovsky oak because long ago it was planted by the great Russian general, Alexander Suvorov.

Many years ago, during the Russian-Turkish war, Suvorov's troops crushed the Turkish army and were returning to Russia through Moldova (in the eighteenth century Moldova was called Bessarabia). Before they began to ferry across the big river Dniester in Moldova, they stopped for a picnic. For several months Suvorov's soldiers rested on the hill. They were exhausted after many long battles with the Turks. However they returned home victoriously and deserved to have a good vacation. General Suvorov had a good time here also. His camp was built near the village in the lovely, sunny valley. He and his soldiers enjoyed the warm sun, the tepid waters of the river, tasty fruits and vegetables, the fresh air of the forest, the beautiful village women, and the hospitality of its people. Some of them married local girls and remained in the village.

Suvorov was so impressed with the people's hospitality and appreciation that when it was time to leave, he decided to do something significant for them to remember that the Russian troops saved this small country from Turkish invaders. He was a generous, kind man and planted the oak on the hill where his army had rested.

"Grow big here, young oak tree," he said, "and let the people remember us, the soldiers that defeated the invaders and brought such desirable freedom and peace to all living in this small, wonderful country."

Then he took a bucket of water from the Dniester river and poured it on the ground where he planted his tree. After that Suvorov mounted a white horse with a golden saddle and signaled to his soldiers to ferry across the river. Old and young people and children from the village gathered on the riverbanks to say goodbye, and they watched the troops disappear from their view. Now, in this wonderful valley, where more than two centuries ago Suvorov's army found a hospitable place to rest, wheat and corn fields stand in golden bloom.

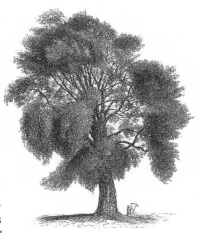

Andrew looked at the amazing Herculean oak. Each of its leaves was like a masterpiece of Nature. Each looked like a delicate, expansive jewel in gold and bronze, and suddenly he understood that only Nature is capable of creating this special art, and this art is inaccessible to us, people.

Let us listen to her tender music and then we will understand the eternal language of the forest—of the trees. We'll hear the delicate sound of trembling leaves and the songs of happy birds. We'll see with new eyes the rich colors of fading leaves in autumn, crystal trees in the winter snow, talkative pine groves, and flowers in the spring in this mysterious silence under the oak's shadow.

The tree's branches were slightly moving under a light breeze. The powerful oak was standing as a soldier, ready to thwart any attack from a newcomer with bad intentions. The clean fragrance of warm leaves hung in the air. The leaves had been rustling in the light wind. It seemed to me that they tried eagerly to tell everyone how wonderful the forest was in all four seasons of the year; and about Suvorov's oak, Hercules, and about his remarkable friends, loving passionately this amazing treasure of the earth and carefully guarding her fabulous green attire.

When I was leaving, at the end of the village on the shore of the Dniester river, three tall poplars peacefully murmured a good-bye and stood quietly in their miraculous splendor. It seemed that they stepped out of an ancient myth about Phaeton, the son of Phoebus, god of the sun, and Clymene, a nymph. He asked his father to do an impossible thing: to appear in the sky instead of the god of the sun. He was allowed to drive his chariot across the sky, but it was too much for the young man. He lost direction in the sky and couldn't control the powerful winged horses that pulled the chariot. Everything was on fire in the sky and on the earth and could be destroyed.

Then the god Zeus threw the sparkling lightning with his thunderbolt and extinguished the fire—but not before the fire had killed the young man. Phaeton fled into the air with the curls on his head still burning, and like a falling star he tumbled in flames from the sun's chariot into the waves of the river Eridanos (Eridanus, now the river Po), far away from his motherland. There water nymphs buried him on the banks of the river.

Deeply mourning, Phaeton's father, the god of the sun, covered his face with a black shawl and did not appear in the blue sky all day. His mother, Clymene, and his three sisters, the Heliades, sat near his grave and wept on the riverbank. They remained weeping and murmuring until their feet took root in the earth. Great gods turned the crying Heliades into poplar trees. These three poplar trees remain kneeling above the river, with their tears falling into clear water. They never stop throwing their tears into the river, where they solidify. In the sunlight their tears of sap have a golden color and turn into transparent, yellow amber.

When Pliny wrote his *Natural History*, he doubted the story of the poplar, which was told also by Ovid in his poetic metamorphoses. Maybe he was right because the most popular version is that amber was made 50 millions years ago from the resinous matters of only one variety of pine tree, *Pinus succinfera*. It grew from the early Eocene period until today in the northern part of Europe, the area covered by the Baltic Sea, which includes Scandinavian countries and the Baltic states of Lithuania, Latvia, Estonia, and Poland.

Would you like to determine what tree corresponds to your birth date? Use this calendar from the book *The Celtic Tree Calendar, Your Tree Sign and You* by Swiss writer Michael Vescolli. This book was published in English translation in 1999 by British publisher Souvenir Press, Ltd., and Rosemary Dear (English translation). I would like to thank Souvenir Press, Ltd. for permission to reprint information from their book.

Your Tree Sign

From *The Celtic Tree Calendar Your Tree Sign and You*
by Swiss writer Michael Vescolli

Oak		**Olive**
21 Mar		23 Sept
22 – 31 Mar	Hazel	24 Sept – 3 Oct
1 –10 April	Rowan	4 – 13 Oct
11 – 20 April	Maple	14 – 23 Oct
21 – 30 April	Walnut	24 Oct – 11 Nov
1 – 14 May	**Poplar**	
15 – 24 May	Chestnut	12 – 21 Nov
25 May – 3 June	Ash	22 Nov – 1 Dec
4 – 13 June	Hornbeam	2 – 11 Dec
14 – 23 June	Fig	12 – 21 Dec

Birch		**Beech**
24 June		22 Dec
25 June – 4 July	Apple	23 Dec – 1 Jan
5 – 14 July	Fir	2 – 11 Jan
15 – 25 July	Elm	12 – 24 Jan
26 July – 4 Aug	Cypress	25 Jan – 3 Feb
5 – 13 Aug	**Poplar**	4 – 8 Feb
14 –23 Aug	Cedar	9 – 18 Feb
24 Aug – 2 Sept	Pine	19 – 29 Feb
3 – 12 Sept	Willow	1 – 10 Mar
13 – 22 Sept	Lime	11 – 20 Mar
	Yew	
	3 – 11 Nov	

You can use also the following chart where I name these trees based on my experience and my impression in dealing with these powerful creatures of Mother Nature.

Apple, the tree of Beauty and Love	December 23–January 1 June 25–July 4
Fir, the tree of Independent Spirit	January 2–January 11 July 5–July 14
Elm, the tree of Fairness and Solidarity	January 12–January 24 July 15–July 25
Cypress, the tree of Freedom and Recognition	January 25–February 3 July 26–August 4
Poplar, the tree of Moderation and Doubt	February 4–February 8 May 1–May 14 August 5–August 13
Cedar, the tree of Achievement and Nobility	February 9–February 18 August 14–August 23
Pine, the tree of Modesty and Wisdom	February 19–February 29 August 24–September 2
Willow, the tree of Humanity and Intuition	March 1–March 10 September 3–September 12
Lime, the tree of Sensitivity and Satisfaction	March 11–March 20 September 13–September 22
Hazelnut, the tree of Ambition and Performance	March 22–March 31 September 24–October 3
Rowan, the tree of Harmony and Perfection	April 1–April 10 October 4–October 13
Maple, the tree of Determination	April 11–April 20 October 14–October 23
Walnut, the tree of Passion and Power	April 21–April 30 October 24–November 11
Chestnut, the tree of Honesty and Quality	May 15–May 24 November 12–November 21

Ash, the tree of Flexibility and Healing

Hornbeam, the tree of Loyalty and
    Protection

Fig, the tree of Comfort and Balance

Oak, the tree of Vitality and Power

Birch, the tree of Light and Beginning

Olive, the tree of Happiness and Prosperity

Beech, the tree of Necessity and Patience

Yew, the tree of Survival and Death

May 25–June 3
November 22–December 1

June 4–June 13
December 2–December 11

June 14–June 23
December 12–December 21

March 21
(spring vernal equinox)

June 24
(summer solstice)

September 23
(autumn vernal equinox)

December 22
(winter solstice)

November 3–November 11

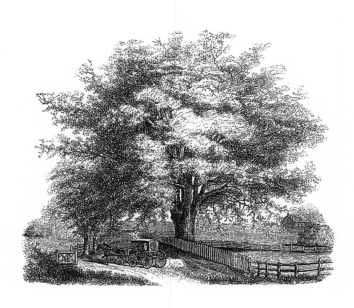

$\mathcal{T}$his is interesting to know:

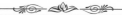

- In federal reserves and national parks, the United States and Canadian governments have the largest area of protected forests in the world—greater than Russia, Germany, Sweden, Finland, Brazil, and the United Kingdom combined. Canada has nearly 86.5 million acres of protected forests, the largest protected area in the world. Canada's area of protected forests is equivalent to the size of Germany. National parks in 49 states of the United States account for another 83 million acres (33.6 million hectare) of forest and no forest land.

- North America's forests are abundant and growing. The forests in the United States and Canada make 15 percent of the Earth's forest cover. The coniferous trees of the Pacific Northwest, the broadleaf forests of Appalachia, and the mixed forests of the United States South support a large number of diverse species of wildlife.

- According to the U.S. Department of Agriculture Forest Service, forest planting in the United States currently averages about one million hectares a year.

- The average North American uses 18 cubic feet (½ cubic meter of wood) and 749 pounds (340 kilograms) of paper per year, equal to a 100-foot (30 meter) tree.

- The single oldest living tree on Earth is a twisted bristle-cone pine named "Methuselah." It grows in the White Mountains of California. It is 4,723 years old and there are other pines in the area that are nearly as old. These trees have been growing since the time when Egyptians were building the pyramids.

- The tallest tree in the world is a 367.5-foot (112 meters) redwood in Montgomery Woods State Preserve in northern California. This tree is 63.5 feet (19.4 meters) taller than the Statue of Liberty and over twice as high as Niagara Falls.

- More than 5,000 products are made from trees: houses, fences, furniture, baseball bats, books, newspapers, tires, cellophane, fabric rayon, and explosives.

- Wood fiber derived from the trees and called cellulose is one of ingredients in production of ice cream, toothpaste, and shampoo.

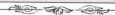

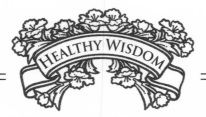

Each disease has its own healing herb.

—*Russian proverb*

Keep a green tree in your heart and perhaps the singing bird will come.

—*Chinese proverb*

Tall oaks from little acorns grow.

—*Anonymous*

It is remarkably pleasant occupation, to lie on one's back in a forest and look upwards! It seems that you are looking into a bottomless sea, that it is stretching out far and wide below you, that the trees are not rising from the earth but, as if they were the roots of enormous plants, are descending or falling steeply into those lucid, glassy waves.

—*Ivan Turgenev (1818–1883), Russian writer*

. . . because the Forest will always be there . . . and anybody who is friendly with bears can find it.

—*A. A. Milne (1882–1956), English poet and writer*

We all travel the Milky Way together, trees and men; but it never occurred to me until this stormy day, while swinging in the wind, that trees are travelers, in the ordinary sense.

—*John Muir (1838–1914), Scottish-born American naturalist*

. . . old Indian teaching was that it is wrong to tear loose from its place on the earth anything that may be growing there. It may be cut off, but it should not be uprooted. The trees and grass have spirits.

—*Wooden Leg, 19th-century American (Cheyenne) warrior*

I like trees because they seem more resigned to the way they have to live than other things do.

—*Willa Cather (1876–1947), American novelist*

Those beeches and smooth limes—there was something enervating in the very sight of them; but the strong knotted old oaks had no bending languor in them—the sight of them would give a man some energy.

—*George Eliot [Mary Anne Evans] (1819–1880), English novelist*

The wonder is that we can see these trees and not wonder more.

—*Ralph Waldo Emerson (1803–1882), American essayist and poet*

Chapter 13

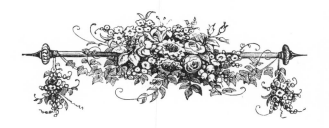

As Isis, So Is Mama . . .

She existed before time began. Time was one of Her children!

—*Nancy Blair,* The Book of Goddesses

As Isis, the Egyptian goddess; Kali, the Indian goddess; Tara, the Mother Goddess of Tibet and India; Greek goddesses Hera, Demeter, and Gaia; and the tender and powerful Mother Nature are archetypes of the Mother, so is Mama. Thus, we all are. We are the sense of the Universe's existence. We conceive, give the birth to, and hold a new life, a new generation.

The mother archetype drives women to be generous; to nourish, provide, and care for others; to nurture body, soul, and spirit. Just as a pregnant woman radiates love, beauty, and blissfulness, so do all "mamas" pass those traits along to their children and others whose lives they touch.

The mother archetype influences men and women alike, at first by building them cell by cell and then by guiding them gently yet firmly and fully into their own lives with all the wisdom she bestows upon them.

So what do you do first to live in this wisdom? Where do you begin and how do you become a wise guide for yourself and your family? How do you organize yourself at first to be a good achiever? I hope the following remedies without herbs, but with healthy thoughts, will help you answer these questions.

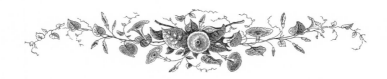

$\mathcal{F}$ifteen secrets of success for all moms who work at home or away from home

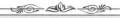

1. Style of Thinking

Different people think in different ways. The relation of thinking to being, how you think, is everything: Always be positive, punctual, considerate, and confident in yourself. Don't be negative; you can lose. As you know, positive energy creates and builds us. Negative energy destroys us.

2. In Search of Yourself

Determine your goal and dreams. Write down your specific goals, decide upon your true dreams, and develop a plan to achieve them. Then just go for it. Don't listen to others who want to discourage you. Trust your soul.

3. Preparation and Action

Prepare and begin acting without any delay. Do everything you can today. Don't leave your decision until tomorrow. Goals are nothing without action. Don't be afraid to get started now. Just do what you plan. Johann Wolfgang von Goethe, a German poet, said once, "It is not enough only to wish. You must act." Actions always speak louder than words.

4. Educate Yourself

An old expression teaches us "Live a century, learn a century." Take some additional courses at college. Read "know-how" and "do-it-yourself" books. Absorb to your benefit good examples from stories about people who have reached their goals and are successful. Perfect yourself and your knowledge. Cultivate your talent or gift. Get training and acquire new skills, if you feel a need for them. Your efforts will be repaid a hundredfold.

5. Be Self-Confident, Persistent, Consistent, and Fearless and Work Hard

Success is a long marathon. It is not a fast sprinter's distance. Success doesn't happen overnight. It happens overnight only in fairy tales, but don't get discouraged. Never give up what you started already. Sooner or later a right beginning will bring you a bountiful basket of good achievements.

6. Analysis and Consideration

Learn to analyze all details and think them over. Our life and everything we do is like a big oil painting by a great artist. Put together ideas, facts, and details. Every small detail makes a big difference and adds to a whole picture. Learn from your mistakes and setbacks. Don't ignore them; they are a good lesson for the future.

7. People, Attention, Time, and Money

Value your time and money, but remember people should always come first. Focus your attention on these matters. Don't permit other people or things to distract or confuse you. Beware of negative environments and irritating or manipulating people. Defend yourself by keeping an "arm's length" distance or just ignore them. Make friends with good, decent people. Search for those who stimulate your interest and respect.

8. Experiments, Innovation, Changes, and Challenges

Don't be afraid to experiment, implement innovation, and head for challenges and changes to the better life. Be different. Following the crowd is annoying and a sure path to mediocrity and intellectual sluggishness.

9. Communication Skills, Respect, and Effectiveness

Communicate and deal with other people effectively and respectfully. No person is a lonely star but a part of a big constellation of others. Learn to understand and motivate others in a positive way. You will usually get a good response.

10. Combination for Success

Be kind. Be loyal. Be pleasant and friendly. Do the best you can. Help and respect other people. Take responsibility for your actions and your life. Don't blame others for your failures; this attitude shows your weakness. See the root of your problem in yourself at first. It will show how strong you are. This combination leads to success.

11. Faith and Hope

Remember an ancient wisdom "*Dum Spiro, Spero*," (Latin) which means "While I breathe, I hope." Hope is like a shining lighthouse in the azure-blue ocean of life. There we fight for our survival every day. Life proves that only the strongest and the best will be able to swim so far to the shore and reach their big goals. Be one of them! Believe in this truth; thus you may understand: "Faith is an understanding of life and the recognition of duties following this understanding," said Russian writer Leo Tolstoy.

12. Standards

Put in front of you only high standards in everything as your great motivation. This way you will accomplish a lot in your life. If your life is based on low standards, you'll achieve very little.

13. Be kind and reasonable

By doing kind acts, we strengthen ourselves. Being reasonable, we do good deeds automatically which leads us to success in the end.

14. Credo: Honesty, Dignity, and Conscience

Honesty and dignity are not a safe shield of self-defense, but convey to others our values in life. Our conscience is our guide in the search for the best in us. It is our internal judge that determines if our actions, words, or attitudes are reprehensible or merit censure.

15. Be Fair, Dependable, Truthful, and Reliable

Take the courage, liberty, and responsibility for your life, your actions, and your family. Otherwise, numbers 1–14 won't matter at all.

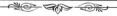

Mama's memos about children

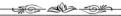

- All children are bright and smart. They are the most amazing miracles given to you. They are beautiful, talented, and kindhearted.

- You love them with all your heart, even if they give you a hard time sometimes. But what are mothers for? The answer is simple: Forgive no matter what, because you and no one else brought them into this wonderful world.

- Never forget that you are the mother. Accept this title with the big responsibility which comes with it. Moms are like apple trees, blooming with delicate rose-white spring flowers. These flowers turn one day into fresh green apples. These are our children, sitting happily in our arms (branches) until we give them a chance to fly high in life.

- Feel obligated to give children a right direction before they will sail independently. It's your sacred duty. Know quite well that they will demand too much from you. They always test you too.

- Should you spoil them? Yes, you should, but do it in a smart and reasonable way because nobody will do it so lovingly as you'll do as their mother. You gave birth to them and the right to live on the planet Earth.

- Sort out your priorities and you'll discover that your No.1 obligation is to create for your children a comfortable home that they will respect, will want to be part of, and will desire to live in.

- Think over and over again about your great responsibility to be the mother and how important it is to provide your children with a warm home and a happy, encouraging atmosphere. If you are able to do it, they will never forget where they came from.

- All children prefer their parents to be firm with them, but they will never tell you that. However, it makes them feel more secure and confident if you keep your word.

- Detect when your children form bad habits. Don't miss these, especially in the early ages. At this stage you'll be able to help them efficiently. You can explain to them the difference between bad and good things, positive and negative acts. This approach will help you prevent them from destroying their lives in the future.

- Put yourself on high alert during the first seven years of the lives of your children. These years are very special. This is a very important time when they learn, with your help, the basics of life and how to be a good human being. It is crucial that we teach our children wholesome values they will carry with them through the rest of their days.

- Always tell them how good they are. Never let them down. Don't intimidate them or make them shy.

- If your children do something wrong, talk to them quietly in private. Explain in a kind manner their mistakes. Always do that no matter how angry you are at the moment. Keep your anger to yourself.

- Never correct them in front of others, especially their friends. They want to look good in other people's eyes. Your children will notice how you behave yourself and will appreciate it.

- Keep your discontent to yourself if you disagree with you husband on how you should raise your children. Never argue with him in front of them. It makes them feel unhappy and unsafe when their parents, who are supposed to be strong and powerful adults, cannot find common ground.

- Let your children see a harmony in your actions and your good relationship with your spouse. They will grow to be happy and confident people.

- Never nag your children again and again about their mistakes. Don't threaten them with punishment or say that the mistake is equal to a sin. They become confused. It upsets their sense of values.

- Be loving, kind, and protective, but don't protect them from consequences. They need to see and learn the painful way once in a while.

- Don't promise your children too much as an impulse of your good mood. Be fair and reasonable with your promises. Try to keep your word no matter what. Remember, they'll feel very disappointed and greatly let down if the promises are broken.

- Don't demand explanations from your children. They will never explain themselves the way you do. They will not always be precise and accurate as you think they should be.

- Forgive your children their bad behavior or bad attitude towards you.

- Don't fight with your children. Don't try to prove your point. Remember that you brought them into the world. Very soon they will stand on the thorny path of life and will try to make something of it. Only you are their first friend, mentor, an aide in each step. Be patient, fair, and resolve everything peacefully so they will have you to depend on.

- Don't be inconsistent in your behavior and actions. That will greatly confuse your children and they will lose their respect for you.

- Don't scream at your children if they do something unexpected and wrong. They will get angry and will want to do wrong things again.

- Even if you feel it is "below your dignity," have the courage to apologize to your children. An honest apology will gain their respect and love and will make them feel happy and warm towards you. Their attitude will come as a nice surprise and a beautiful gift to you.

- You may think highly about yourself, that you are a great mother, that you accomplished a lot in your life, and became a good person, but don't ever tell that to your children. Don't ever suggest that you are perfect and fully accomplished. If you do, it will give them a big shock when they discover one day that you are neither.

- Show them sincerely your respect and they will respect you in return.

- Attract their attention in a smart, innovative way. Joke and chat with your children and they will believe in you, love you, and support you.

- Never use words of bravado when you want to tell your children about your personal or somebody else's achievements in the past. They will spot right away when you try too hard to convince them of something.

- Show by example the way you act from your heart. Children are excellent observers, better than we think. They absorb everything, good or bad like a sponge. If they like what you do, they will duplicate your good endeavors. They will duplicate the bad ones too, if you let them.

- Remember, children are like beautiful flowers. They are fragile, confused, loving, and delicate. Sometimes they are not fair and even rude. Don't take to your heart their "downs."

- Encourage your children to reach for the stars, dream, and be the best they can be.

- Albert Einstein said once, "If you want your children to be brilliant, tell them fairy tales. If you want them to be very brilliant, tell them even more fairy tales." Make your children wonder. Teach them that good actions will always give them strength and inspire the same in others.

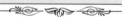

Can you imagine the happiness of a young hero of an ancient folk tale from the far North? He entered the Valley of Flowers, saved the lives of his father and many other people, and changed a malicious witch to a beautiful, kind girl. Then he married her and lived happily ever after. I heard it from Grandma in my childhood and told it many times to my children to show them that good actions will always give them strength, confidence, and the desire to do something good with their life.

Valley of Flowers

*O*nce far away up north a husband and wife lived in one tribe. The husband went hunting and brought home birds to feed his family. His wife took care of their four deer, sewed new clothes, and maintained the house. They had a lot of children born, but all of them died—one after another.

One day early in the morning the husband went hunting again. While he was absent, his wife gave birth to another son. His face looked like a full moon. His eyes shone like two stars. His delicate skin had a pink glow like a spring dawn. His mother gave him a bath with salty water, and his skin was healthy and smooth. Herbal teas and tasteful vegetable meals also made the boy strong and gave him a great endurance in case something bad happened.

Much time passed, but the boy's father didn't come back home from hunting. Days passed one after another. The son grew big and fast in the father's absence.

Finally the boy decided that his time had come to go and look for his father. One day he made a bow from the branches of a young birch. Then he showed it to his mother and asked her permission to go hunt and try his luck to find his father. His mother gave him her blessings.

For the first time in his life the young boy left his parents' house and went to the unknown and mysterious forest. He didn't have any food with him, so he had to feed himself with game birds that he shot during the day. At night he fell asleep under a cedar tree. In the morning he washed up in the mountain spring and went further and further.

Once at night a terrible scream woke him up. The young hunter got scared. He bent his bow and stood ready to defend himself. Suddenly he heard a woman laughing. He thought the sound came from the top of the cedar tree where he stood. He looked at the summit of the tree and saw a snowy owl. This was the owl waking him up in the middle of the night and making fun of him.

The young man became angry and directed the arrow towards the owl, but the owl flew to another tree and said, "OK, brother Ula, don't be angry. Just remember where you are going and what you want to do, and I will help you. From this time on, you'll sleep during the day. At night you'll go search for your father. I can tell you for sure that your father is alive, but he was bewitched by a vicious sorceress. You must save him, mustn't you?"

The owl flew through the dense forest three nights. Ula followed her step by step. Three days the owl sat in the hollow of a tree, and Ula slept under the same tree. On the fourth night the owl said to Ula, "Now we'll soon be in the sorceress' charmed place. She'll try to put you to sleep, but you shouldn't fall asleep because you'll lose control, and you will not be able to save your father. Fill your pockets with stones and small twigs. Put them under your body when you feel drowsy, and then you can guess what you have to do. I'll be close by; don't worry."

At midnight Ula came to a beautiful, sparkling green meadow. He heard a ringing of cymbals and a tinkling of bells. A young girl's voice was singing a melodic song. Every flower emanated its radiance. Ula could see a yellow thin strip between all flowers of the meadow.

Ula could hardly keep his eyes opened. He lay down on the emerald grass and suddenly he recalled what the owl told him. He gathered stones and twigs and placed them under his body. However, an invisible girl continued to sing her beautiful songs, each one sweeter than the last. The bells continued to tinkle, and the cymbals continued ringing. Ula's head fell heavily into the grass, but the stones and twigs were uncomfortable. He opened his eyes and exclaimed, "Who does the singing there? Who prevents me from my peaceful sleep with these songs?"

"This is me," responded a voice of an invisible girl.

"Who are you? Show up."

"Now I cannot show up. You can find me only at sunrise."

"Tell me, how can I find you?" Ula asked.

"Do you see the yellow strip? Come close by at sunrise and you will see me," answered the girl.

Then Ula heard the outcry of the owl, and he understood that the time had come to catch the sorceress. He jumped back on his feet and ran to the yellow strip. The bells and cymbals were clanking with difficulty. Ula approached the yellow strip and saw a beautiful shining woman's sash. He grabbed it with both hands, and a girl of unspeakable beauty appeared in front of him. She wore a yellow dress. The youth looked at her and forgot why he had come here. The owl gave him again a loud outcry.

"Why didn't you wait until sunrise had come? Why didn't you listen to me?" the girl asked Ula frowning.

"Because now you are powerless," Ula replied. "You will not bewitch me and I am not afraid of you. Tell me where my father is and what you did to him."

The girl stood silent in front of him. The owl's outcry resounded again. "Tell me immediately where my father is or I'll tear down your sash and you'll lose your power!" Ula demanded in anger, ripping her sash from her dress.

"Your father is here, but he is blind. He looked at me at sunrise. Anyone who looks at me at the daybreak becomes blind from my beauty and my bright dress," the girl replied. "Give me back my sash and I'll bring you to your father."

"No, first you bring me to my father, and then I'll see if I will give you back your sash," Ula continued.

The bells began tinkling and cymbals ringing again. One red flower opened up. It rocked and then it threw all its petals to the ground. In a blink of an eye, a hunter appeared in front of Ula. This hunter looked like him, Ula.

"I don't see you, the sorceress," he said. "Let me touch your sash; it will give me my life back."

"Your son came after you," replied the girl. "I give you your freedom because of him, but you will still be blind."

The hunter was happy anyway. His cheeks became wet from his tears. But the next minute the owl gave her outcry again. Ula looked at the valley and saw myriad flowers there. He guessed that all those flowers were the misfortunate hunters who had been charmed by the sorceress the same as his father had.

"Well, what you want to give me is not enough, smart girl. Liberate all the hunters you charmed," Ula said. "I don't want even one flower to be left on your meadow."

The sorceress became very angry, but she couldn't do anything. She gave a sign, and all flowers opened up at once. They rocked and threw their petals on the ground. The stems began to grow and in several minutes 77 hunters stood in front of Ula. All of them were blind. The owl gave an outcry again, and Ula crumpled the yellow sash with one fast clenching of his fist. Then he burned the sash and put the ashes in a wooden cup.

The owl gave an outcry again, and the young man came up to his father and rubbed his eyes with the ash. His father began to see again. Ula did the same with all 77 hunters and all of them gained their sight back. They were very happy to be free. They thanked Ula for saving their lives and giving them back their healthy eyes.

But the next minute the owl-friend cried again. Ula understood that something was not finished yet. He looked at the girl. She was sitting on the grass, an unspeakable beauty in the yellow shining dress, and she was crying.

"Why do you cry? I see now you are not a malicious witch but a normal girl. You are so beautiful that I have fallen in love with you," said Ula. "Do you know what? Promise to be good and I will take you with us, and I'll marry you. We'll live together and I'll be a good husband to you."

The end of this fairy tale was happy. Ula, his father, and the girl returned home together. Ula's mother met them with a big smile and a warm hospitality that only she could provide as a real mother. She liked the girl at first sight. There was a big, merry wedding, and all 77 hunters were invited with their families. They celebrated seven days and seven nights.

And from that time on hunters are not scared to go back to the Valley of Flowers because now hundreds of red flowers grow there, blossom, and dance gracefully at sunrise. They murmur and share the peoples' secrets with the wind, and sing marvelous songs, known only to them alone.

When I think about this old folk tale, I feel that it is surprisingly compatible with the real life we lead. Albert Einstein said, not by chance, that if we want our children to be brilliant, we should read them fairy tales. He said so from his observations and his own experience. We can trust his suggestion; he was a brilliant man and a genius scientist himself. Perhaps his mother read him a lot of fairy tales.

I believe we must find time in our busy lives to read to our children as much as we can—good children's literature, kind and wise stories, folk tales and fairy tales. As all mothers do, I am sure if we "put" anything good in our children by planting fine "seeds" from the first day of their appearance on Earth, it will give great results in the future. Our children will lead healthy lives, and not "thorny paths," and they will not get hurt easily, if they will choose good actions, and inspire the same in others.

Doesn't the Valley of Flowers remind you too of our everyday life and the fascinating world around that we explore all the time? The place where we and our children share love, joy and appreciation for each other, and the great satisfaction of knowing we should continue our life journey with the best intentions we can?

Our life, our Valley of Flowers, is where millions of peoples' destinies grow and blossom like flowers, dance gracefully at sunrise, and murmur with the wind. Some of these flowers and their neighbors—herbs, trees, fruits, and vegetables—can enhance our health and emotions. Respect them and take advantage of how they can help you and others.

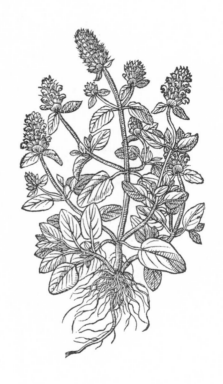

Chapter 14

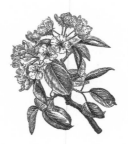

Nature's Green Clinic:
Useful Herbs, Plants, Fruits
and Vegetables

Medicine is an art to imitate the healing power of nature.

*Hippocrates (c.460-c.377 B.C.), Greek physician
and the "Father of Medicine."*

This chapter charts the healing power of our green friends, used in remedies in this book, and how they can be our lifesavers. They come from centuries of people's wisdom and from flora of the earth—an endless treasure of natural healers. Even the most primitive tribes on Earth knew medicinal characteristics of herbs and how to use them. In search of food, human beings observed the faultless instincts of animals, saving themselves with green plants, and they began to recognize the medicinal properties of herbs.

Humans have long studied about how to find and use herbs. One of the important precepts of Hippocrates doctrine was based on the "the healing power of nature," or in Latin, *vis mediatrix naturae.* Theophrastus, Greek philosopher and a student of Aristotle and Dioscorides (circa 372-287 B.C.), wrote *Medicinal Matters*, in which he prescribed the experiences of ancient Egyptians, Assyrians, and Babylonians and the use of 600 plants or herbs. His book was translated into Latin with the name *Materia Medica* and served as a guide to doctors and pharmacists for 15 centuries. From that time, Latin names of herbs have become well known and used throughout European countries, Russia, and almost everywhere in the world. Names of herbs, trees, and other plants are given in English and Latin versions.

Chapter 1: Rose Hips Tea Party

Rose hips – *Rosa canina*

Chapter 2: "Even the Badger Knows…"

Almond – *Amygdalis dulcis*
Aloe – *Aloe vera*
Barley – *Hordeum vulgare*
Beet – *Beta vulgaris*
Black radish – *Raphanus sativus*
Cabbage – *Brassica oleracea*
Carrot – *Daucus carota*
Garlic – *Allium sativum*
Ginger – *Zingiber officinale*
Olive (oil) – *Olea europaea*
Onion – *Allium cepa*
Peat moss – *Sphagnum*
Pine. Stone Pine (nuts) – *Pinus pinea*
Pomegranate – *Punica granatum*
Walnut – *Juglans regia*

Chapter 3: A Healthy Spirit Lives in a Healthy Body

Almond, almond oil – *Amygdalis dulcis*
Apple – *Malus domestica*
Apricot (dried, or apricot kernel oil) – *Prunus armeniaca*
Beet – *Beta vulgaris*
Black tea – *Camellia sinensis*
Burdock – *Arctium lappa*
Cabbage – *Brassica oleracea*
Calendula – *Calendula officinalis*
Chamomile – *Matricaria chamomilla/ M. recutita*

Coffee (beans) – *Coffea arabica*
Dandelion – *Taraxacum officinale*
Dried grape (raisin) – *Vitis vinifera*
Evening primrose oil – *Oenothera biennis*
Garden radish – *Raphanus sativis*
Garlic – *Allium sativum*
Grape, Grapeseed oil – *Vitis vinifera*
Grapeseed oil – *Vitis vinifera*
Lemon – *Citrus limon*
Olive (oil) – *Olea europaea*
Plum – *Prunus domestica*
Potato – *Solanum tuberosum*
Prune (dried plum) – *Prunus domestica*
Rose hips oil – *Rosa canina*
Tomato – *Solanum lycopersicum*
Turnip – *Brassica rapa*
Walnut – *Juglans regia*
Wheat germ oil – *Triticum durum*

Chapter 4: Stop Sneezes And Sniffles and Stifle a Cold

Anise – *Pimpinella anisum*
Apple – *Malus domestica*
Beet – *Beta vulgaris*
Birch – *Betula alba*
Black currant – *Ribes nigrum*
Black elder, elderberry – *Sambucus nigra*
Black elder, Siberian elder – *Sambucus nigra*
Blackthorn – *Prunus spinosa*
Bogbean – *Menyanthes trifoliata*
Buckthorn – *Rhamnus frangula*
Calendula – *Calendula officinalis*
Carrot – *Daucus carota*

Centaury (an old World herb)
– *Centaurium erythraea*
Chamomile – *Matricaria chamimilla/
M. recutita*
Cherry – *Prunus cerasus*
Coltsfoot – *Tussilago farfara*
Elecampane – *Unula helenium*
English oak – *Quercus robur*
Fennel – *Foeniculum officinale*
Feverfew – *Tanacetum parthenium*
Garlic – *Allium sativum*
German golden locks – *Gnaphalium
avenarium*
Greater celandine – *Chelidonium majus*
Hawthorn – *Crataegus monogyna/
C. laevigata*
Heartsease – *Viola tricolor*
Lemon – *Citrus limon*
Licorice – *Glycyrrhiza glabra*
Linden – *Tilia europea*
Lungwort – *Pulmonaria officinalis*
Marsh cudweed – *Gnaphalium uliginosum*
Marshmallow – *Althaea officinalis*
Mint – *Mentha*
Mullein – *Verbascum thapsus*
Nettle (stinging) – *Urtica dionica*
Oat straw – *Avena sativa*
Onion – *Allium cepa*
Orange – *Citrus aurantium*
Peppermint – *Mentha piperita*
Poppy – *Papaver rhoeas*
Potato – *Solanum tuberosum*
Raspberry – *Rubus idaeus*
Red bilberry – *Vaccinium myrtillis*
Rose hips – *Rosa canina*
Sage – *Salvia officinalis*
St. John's Wort – *Hypericum perforatum*
Strawberry – *Fragaria vesca*
Sunflower oil – *Helianthus annuus*
Sweet brier, Eglantine –*Rosa rubiginosa*
Tangerine – *Citrus reticulata*
Thyme – *Thymus*

Vanilla (extract) – *Vanilla planifolia*
White oak – *Quercus alba*
Wild marjoram – *Origanum vulgare*
Willow – *Salix alba*
Wood betony – *Betonica officinalis*
(in Europe used to treat about 30
diseases. W.b. is not commonly
used in the U.S.A.)

Chapter 5:
A Sickness of the 21st Century

Agrimony – *Agrimonia eupatoria*
Apple – *Malus domestica*
Apricot – *Prunus armeniaca*
Birch – *Betula verrucosa*
Black currant – *Ribes nigrum*
Black tea – *Camelia sinensis*
Blueberry – *Vaccinium vitis idaea*
Burdock – *Arctium lappa*
Cabbage – *Brassica oleracea*
Calendula (pot marigold) – *Calendula
officinalis*
Carrot – *Daucus carota*
Celery – *Apium graveolens*
Chamomile – *Matricaria chamomilla/
M.recutita*
Cherry – *Prunus cerasus*
Coffee – *Coffea arabica*
Corn silk – *Zea mays*
Cranberry – *Vaccinium oxycoccus*
Dandelion – *Taraxacum officinale*
Duckweed (aquatic plant) – *Lemna minor*
Eyebright – *Euphrasia officinalis*
Garlic – *Allium sativum*
Gooseberry – *Ribes glossularia*
Greater celandine – *Chelidonium majus*
Heartsease – *Viola tricolor*
Hops – *Humulus lupulus*
Horsetail – *Equisetum arvense*
Jasmine – *Jasminum officinale*
Lemon – *Citrus limon*
Motherwort – *Leonurus cardiaca*

Mountain Ash – *Sorbus*
Nettle – *Urtica dionica*
Oak (bark) – *Quercus robur*
Oat – *Avena sativa*
Olive(oil) – *Olea europaea*
Onion – *Allium cepa*
Orange – *Citrus aurantium*
Parsley – *Petroselinum crispum*
Passionflower – *Passiflora incarnata*
Peony – *Paeonia officinalis*
Peppermint – *Mentha piperita*
Rose hips – *Rosa canina*
Self-Heal – *Prunella vulgaris*
St. John's Wort – *Hypericum perforatum*
Strawberry – *Fragaria vesca*
Valerian – *Valeriana officinalis*
Yarrow – *Achillea millefolium*

Chapter 6: Ourselves, Our Children, Allergens, and Happy Cells

Agrimony – *Agrimonia eupatoria*
Apple – *Malus domestica*
Birch – *Betula verrucosa*
Black currant – *Ribes nigrum*
Burdock (root) – *Arctium lappa*
Calendula – *Calendula officinalis*
Chamomile – *Matricaria recutita*
Cherry – *Prunus cerasus*
Cranberry – *Vaccinium oxycoccus*
Dandelion (root) – *Taraxacum officinale*
Elecampane – *Unula helenium*
Gentian – *Gentiana lutea*
Gooseberries – *Ribes glossularia*
Heartsease – *Viola tricolor*
Horsetail – *Equisetum arvense*
Juniper – *Juniperus communis*
Licorice – *Glycyrrhiza glabra*
Licorice – *Glycyrrhiza spp.*
Nettle – *Urtica dionica*
Oak – *Quercus robur*
Oat – *Avena sativa*
Peppermint – *Mentha piperita*

Pine – *Pinus sylvestris/ Pinus cembra*
Quince – *Cydonia oblongata*
Rose – *Rosa centifolia, Rosa damascena*
Rose hip – *Rosa canina*
Rye – *Secale cereale*
Sage – *Salvia officinalis*
Strawberry – *Fragaria vesca*
Thyme – *Thymus vulgaris*
Wheat bran – *Triticum durum*
Wild marjoram – *Origanum vulgare*
Yarrow – *Achillea millefolium*

Chapter 7: Clever Remedies to Outsmart Headaches

Black currant – *Ribes nigrum*
Black radish – *Raphanus sativus*
Black tea – *Camellia sinensis*
Burdock – *Arctium lappa*
Cabbage – *Brassica oleracea*
Calendula – *Calendula arvensis*
Calendula – *Calendula officinalis*
Carrot – *Daucus carota*
Chamomile – *Matricaria chamomilla*
Cherry – *Prunus cerasus*
Cinnamon – *Cinnamomum verum*
Cinnamon – *Cinnamomum zeylanicum*
Clover – *Trifolium pratense*
Coffee – *Coffea arabica*
Coltsfoot – *Tussilago farfara*
Cranberry – *Vaccinium oxycoccus*
Dandelion – *Taraxacum officinalis*
Dill – *Anethum graveolens*
Elder – *Sambucus nigra*
Elecampane – *Unula helenium*
Evening primrose/ *Oenothera biennis)*
Feverfew – *Tanacetum parthenium*
Garlic – *Allium sativum*
Geranium – *Pelargonium*
Ginseng – *Panax*
Green bean – *Phaseolus vulgaris*
Green tea – *Camellia sinensis*
Hawthorn – *Crataegus monogyna*

Horehound (leaves and young shoots)
– *Marrubium vulgare*
Horsetail – *Equisetum arvense*
Jasmine – *Jasminum officinale*
Lavender – *Lavandula officinalis*
Lemon – *Citrus limon*
Lemon balm – *Melissa officinalis*
Lime – *Citrus aurantifolia*
Linden – *Tilia europea*
Mint – *Mentha*
Mountain ash – *Sorbus aucuparia*
Onion – *Allium cepa*
Orange – *Citrus aurantium*
Oregano – *Origanum vulgare*
Peppermint – *Mentha piperita*
Pine – *Pinus sylvestris*
Potato – *Solanum tuberosum*
Primrose – *Primula officinalis*
   (*Primrose should not be confused
   with Evening primrose – *Oenothera
   biennis*)
Raspberry – *Rubus idaeus*
Red bell pepper – *Capsicum frutescens*
St. John's Wort – *Hypericum perforatum*
Strawberry – *Fragaria vesca*
Tangerine – *Citrus reticulata*
Thyme – *Thymus*
Tomato – *Solanum lycopersicum*
Valerian – *Valeriana officinalis*

Chapter 8: Sleeping Beauty

Almond – *Amygdalis dulcis*
Apple – *Malus domestica*
Birch – *Betula alba*
Black currant – *Ribes nigrum*
Bogbean, marsh trefoil – *Menyanthes
   trifoliata*
Buckthorn – *Rhamnus frangula*
Caraway – *Carum carvi*
Carrot – *Daucus carota*
Celery – *Apium graveolens*
Chamomile – *Matricaria chamomilla*

Coffee – *Coffea arabica*
Cranberry – *Vaccinium oxycoccus*
Dill – *Anethum graveolens*
Elder – *Sambucus nigra*
Elder (red berries) – *Sambucus racemosa*
Elecampane – *Unula helenium*
Fennel – *Foeniculum vulgare*
Grape – *Vitis vinifera*
Hawthorn – *Crataegus oxyacantha*
Hops – *Humulus lupulus*
Knotgrass (Bird's buckwheat) –
   Poligonum aviculare
Lavender oil – *Lavandula officinalis*
Lemon – Citrus limon
Lemon balm – *Melissa officinalis*
Lily of the Valley – *Convillaria majalis*
Mint – *Mentha*
Mistletoe – *Viscum album*
Motherwort – *Leonurus cardiaca*
Nettle – *Urtica dionica*
Oat – *Avena sativa*
Orange – *Citrus aurantium*
Passionflower – *Passiflora incarnata*
Peppermint – *Mentha piperita*
Pine – *Pinus sylvestris*
Rose hips – *Rosa canina*
Rosemary – *Rosmarinus officinalis*
Rue – *Ruta graveolens*
   (* Caution: It is a good circulatory
   tonic and antispasmodic, but avoid
   using rue during pregnancy.)
St. John's Wort – *Hypericum perforatum*
Sweet clover – (*Melilotus officinalis*)
Thyme – *Thymus serpyllum*
Tomato – *Solanum tuberosum*
Turnip – *Brassica rapa*
Valerian – *Valeriana officinalis*
Vanilla – *Vanilla plantifolia*
Wild lettuce – *Lactuca virosa*
Wild marjoram – *Origanum vulgare*
Yarrow – *Achillea millefolium*

Chapter 9: When Your Head Is Swimming

Blackberry – *Rubus fructicosus*
Buckwheat – *Polygonum fagopyrum*
Calendula – *Calendula officinalis*
Chamomile – *Matricaria chamomilla*
Cinnamon – *Cinnamomum verum*
Cucumber – *Cucumus sativus*
Dill – *Anethum graveolens*
Green peas – *Pisum sativum*
Hawthorn – *Crataegus oxyacantha*
Mint – *Mentha*
Onion – *Allium cepa*
Paprika – *Capsicum frutescens* varieties
Parsley – *Petroselinium sativum*
Peppermint – *Mentha piperita*
Potato – *Solanum tuberosum*
Radish – *Raphanus sativis*
Sage – *Salvia officinalis*
Walnut – *Juglans regia*

Chapter 10: Don't Be Afraid of Good Stress

Apple – *Malus domestica*
Apricot – *Prunus armeniaca*
Black currant – *Ribes nigrum*
Carrot – *Daucus carota*
Cherry – *Prunus cerasus*
Cranberry – *Vaccinium oxycoccus*
Gooseberry – *Ribes grossularia*
Grape – *Vitis vinifera*
Lemon – *Citrus limon*
Linden – *Tilia europea*
Onion – *Allium cepa*
Peach – *Prunus persica*
Pear – *Pyrus communis*
Plum – *Prunus domestica*
Pumpkin – *Cucurbita pepo*
Raspberry – *Rubus idaeus*
Red currant – *Ribes rubrum*
Rose hips – *Rosa canina*

Sage – *Salvia officinalis*
Strawberry – *Fragaria vesca*
Thyme – *Thymus vulgaris*
Walnut – *Juglans regia*
Watermelon – *Citrullus lanatus*

Stimulating aromas:
Anise – *Pimpinella anisum*
Camphor – *Cinnamomum camphora*
Cardamom – *Elettaria cardamomum*
Cinnamon – *Cinnamomum zeylanicum*
Eucalyptus – *Eucalyptus globulus*
Lemon – *Citrus limon*
Nutmeg – *Myristica fragrans*
Peppermint – *Mentha piperita*
Pine – *Pinus nigra*
Rosemary – *Rosemarinus officinalis*

Relaxing aromas:
Bergamot – *Citrus bergamia*
Chamomile – *Matricaria chamomilla*
Cypress – *Cupressus spp.*
Honeysuckle – *Lonicera periclymenum*
Jasmine – *Jasminum officinale*
Juniper – *Juniperus communis*
Lavender – *Lavandula officinalis*
Lemon balm – *Melissa officinalis*
Orange – *Citrus aurantium*
Periwinkle – *Vinca major*
Rose – *Rosa centifolia, Rosa damascena*
Sandalwood – *Santalum album*

Chapter: 11: Trips to the Fairyland

Aloe – *Aloe vera*
Anise – *Pimpinella anisum*
Barley – *Hordeum vulgare*
Black tea – *Camellia sinensis*
Calendula – *Calendula officinalis*
Chamomile – *Matricaria chamomilla*
Coltsfoot – *Tussilago farfara*
Elder – *Sambucus nigra*
Eucalyptus – *Eucalyptus globulus*
Fennel – *Foeniculum vulgare*

Fennel – *Foeniculum vulgare*
Garlic – *Allium sativum*
Geranium – *Pelargonium*
Ginger – *Zingiber officinale*
Grape – *Vitis vinifera*
Grapefruit – *Citrus paradisi*
Green tea – *Camellia sinensis*
Hawthorn – *Crataegus laevigata*
Hawthorn – *Crataegus oxyacantha*
Hawthorn – *Crataegus oxyacantha*
Heartsease – *Viola tricolor*
Heartsease – *Viola tricolor*
Hops – *Humulus lupulus*
Horseradish – *Armoracia rusticana*
Jasmine – *Jasminum officinale*
Laurel – *Laurus nobilis*
Lavender – *Lavandula officinalis*
Lemon – *Citrus limon*
Licorice – *Glycyrrhiza glabra*
Lilac – *Syringia vulgaris*
Lily – *Lilium candidum*
Linden – *Tilia europea*
Mint – *Mentha*
Mustard – *Sinapsis hirta*
Oak – *Quercus*
Onion – *Allium cepa*
Oregano – *Origanum vulgare*
Pine – *Pinus*
Pine – *Pinus sylvestris*
Plantain – *Plantago lanceolata*
Pomegranate – *Punica granatum*
Poplar – *Populus tremula*
Potato – *Solanum tuberosum*
Raspberry – *Rubus idaeus*
Red bilberry – *Vaccinium myrtillis*
Rose – *Rosa centifolia*
Rose – *Rosa centifolia, damascena*
Rose hips – *Rosa canina*
Rosemary – *Rosmarinus officinalis*
Sundew – *Drosera rotundifolia*
Thyme – *Thymus spp.*
Turnip – *Brassica rapa*

Valerian – *Valeriana officinalis*
Walnut – *Juglans regia*
Wild marjoram – *Origanum vulgare*
Wild strawberry – *Fragaria vesca*
Willow – *Salix spp.*

Chapter 12: Dialogue with the Trees of Strength and Everlasting Life

To admire:
Cyclamen flowers – *Cyclamen europaeum*
Magnolia flowers – *Magnolia glauca*

Essential oils:
Birch oil – *Betula*
Eucalyptus oil – *Eucalyptus globulus*
Lavender oil – *Lavandula officinalis*
Linden oil – *Tilia*
Peppermint oil – *Mentha piperita*
Pine oil – *Pinus*

Aloe – *Aloe vera*
Apple – *Malus domestica*
Beech – *Fagus sylvatica*
Birch – *Betula*
Black currant – *Ribes nigrum*
Black Mulberry – *Morus nigra*
Cedar – *Cedrus*
Chestnut – *Castana vesca*
Cranberry – *Vaccinium oxycoccus*
Cypress – *Cupressus*
Elm – *Ulmus*
European Ash – *Fraxinus excelsior*
Fig – *Ficus carica*
Fir – *Abies alba*
Geranium – *Pelargonium*
Hazelnut – *Corylus avellana*
Hornbeam – *Carpinus Americana*
Laurel – *Laurus nobilis*
Lemon – *Citrus limon*
Linden – *Tilia*
Maple – *Acer*

Mountain Ash – *Sorbus*
Mountain Cranberry Tree –
   Arctostaphylos uva-ursi
Nettle – *Urtica dionica*
Oak – *Quercus*
Olive – *Olea europaea*
Pine – *Pinus*
Plantain – *Plantago lanceolata*

Poplar – *Populus*
Red Mulberry – *Morus rubra*
Rose hips – *Rosa canina*
Rowan – *Sorbus aucuparia*
Walnut – *Juglans regia*
Wild marjoram – *Origanum vulgare*
Willow – *Salix*
Yew – *Taxus baccata*

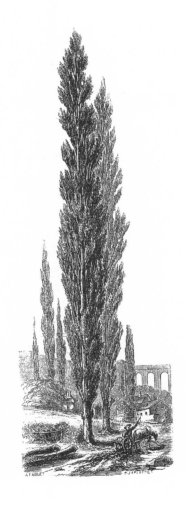

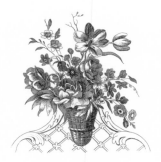

Endnotes

1. Center for Disease Control National Center for Health Statistics, May 27, 2004 (20-page full-text PDF report)

2. Leningrad: "Children's Literature," 1974, 163.

3. *Health, United States, 2002 with Chartbook on Trends in the Health of Americans*, National Center for Health Statistics Report, September 12, 2002.

4. http://www.hhs.gov

5. http://health.gov

6. http://health.gov/healthypeople.

7. JAMA, July 26, 2000, 284 (4), 483-485

8. http://www.mercola.com

9. http://www.healthorg.com

10. Pocket Books, a division of Simon & Schuster, Inc. (New York, 2000).

11. Express Scripts, Inc. www.drugdigest.org

12. www.healthdiscovery.com

13. www.bodybuildingforyou.com

14. http://lungusa.org

15. http://www.health.uab.edu (*U.S. News & World Report* ranked UAB University of Alabama at Birmingham among "America's Best Hospitals")

16. Journal of Allergy and Clinical Immunology, 103:559-62, 1999

17. Advance Data 328

18. Allergy Prevention Center, an in-depth educational and informational online resource for allergy sufferers, www.allergypreventioncenter.com

19. Penelope Ody, (New York: Dorling Kindersley, Inc.), 1993

20. www.eczema.org, reviewed by Dermatologists of the Society Scientific Committee. The National Eczema Society: A Company Limited by Guarantee. Registered in England. Registration No. 2685083.

21. Allergy Prevention Center, www.allergypreventioncenter.com

22. www.headache-helper.com

23. American Council for Headache Education (ACHE), www.achenet.org

24. American Council for Headache Education (ACHE), www.achenet.org

25. The National Migraine Association (MAGNUM), www.migraines.org

26. The National Migraine Association (MAGNUM), www.migraines.org

27. www.headache-helper.com

28. American Council for Headache Education (ACHE), www.achenet.org

29. National Sleep Foundation, www.usdmc.ucdavis.edu

30. www.doctoryourself.com the world's largest health homesteading Web site

31. E. Cheraskin, M.D., D.M.D., *Journal of Orthomolecular Medicine*, 9:1, first quarter 1994, 39-45.

32. Stress Directions, Inc., the Stress Knowledge Company, www.stressdirections.com

33. National Institutes of Health, National Heart, Lung and Blood Institute. Data release for World Asthma Day, May 2001.

34. President's Task Force on Environmental Health Risks and Safety Risks to Children. Asthma and the Environment: A Strategy to Protect Children. Revised May 2000.

35. National Ambulatory Medical Care Survey: 2001 Summary.

36. National Hospital Ambulatory Medical Care Survey: 2002 Emergency Department Summary.

37. U.S. Department of Health and Human Services, "Tracking Healthy People 2010. Section 24–Respiratory Diseases," November 2000, http://www.cdc.gov The national data system is the National Hospital Discharge Survey conducted by the National Center for Health Statistics.

38. http://www.forestinformation.com

39. Research an essential foundation: chapter 14 – Outdoor Recreation in America Parks and Recreation, August 2002. http://uuufindarticles.com

40. If you are interested in yoga, you can read *The Teachings of Integral Yoga* by Sri Swani Satchidananda at www.yogaville.org

41. Henry David Thoreau's first book, *A Week on the Concord and Merrimack Rivers*, 1849, written during his stay at Walden Pond.

42. From John Muir *The Mountains of California*, New York, The Century Co. 1894.

Appendix

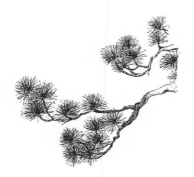

Natural Health Resources

Allergy Health Online Treatment and Prevention
http://allergy.healthcenteronline.com

American Academy of Environmental Medicine
7701 E Kellogg Dr., Ste. 625
Wichita, KS 67207
tel: 316.684.5500
http://www.aaem.com

All Natural Health
A compilation of the best web sites that cater to health-conscious consumers and health-care professionals.
http://allnaturalhealth.us

American Association of Naturopathic Physicians (AANP)
4435 Wisconsin Ave., NW, Ste. 403
Washington, DC 20016
tel: 866.538.2267 ❧ fax: 202.237.8152
http://www.naturopathic.com

American Botanical Council
P.O. Box 144345
Austin, TX 78714
tel: 512.926.4900 ❧ fax:512.916.2245
http://www.herbalgram.org

American Herbal Products Association
8484 Georgia Ave., Ste.370
Silver Springs, MD 20910
tel: 301.588.1171 ❧ fax: 301.588.1174
http://www.ahpa.org

American Herbalists' Guild
141 Nob Hill Road
Cheshire, CT 06410
tel: 203.272.6731 ❧ fax: 203.272.8550

American Holistic Medical Association
P.O. Box 2016, Edmonds, WA 98020
tel: 425.967.0737 ❧ fax: 425.771.9588
http://www.holisticmedicine.org

Association of Natural Medicine Pharmacists
P.O. Box 150727
San Rafael, CA 94915
tel: 415.479.1512 ❧ fax: 415.472.2559
http://www.anmp.org

Bastyr Center for Natural Health
The largest natural health clinic in the State of Washington.
3670 Stone Way N
Seattle, WA 98103
tel: 206.834.4100 ❧ fax: 206.834.4107
http://bastyrcenter.org

Botanical Society of America
P.O. Box 299
St. Louis, MO 63166
tel: 314.577.9566 ❧ fax: 314.577.9515
http://www.botany.org

Centers for Disease Control and Prevention
Public Health Service
US Department of Health and Human Services
1600 Clifton Rd. NE
Atlanta, GA 30333
tel: 404.639.3534 or 800.311.3435 (public inquiries)
http://www.cdc.gov

Citizens for Health
P.O. Box 2260
Boulder, CO 80306
tel: 303.417.0722 or 800.357.2211
fax: 303.417.9378
http://www.citizens.org

Children's Center
www.hopkinschildrens.org

Complementary & Alternative Medicines Institute (CAMI)
University of the Sciences at Philadelphia
600 S. 43rd St.
Philadelphia, PA 19104
tel: 215.596.7598

Green People
World's largest directory of eco-friendly and holistic health products.
http://www.greenpeople.com

Greenpeace USA
702 H Street, NW
Washington, DC 20001
tel: 202.462.1177
— and —
75 Arkansas St.
San Francisco, CA 94107
tel: 415.255.9221
http://www.greenpeace.org

Herb Research Foundation
4140 15th St.
Boulder, CO 80304
tel: 303.449.2265 ❧ fax: 303.449.7849
http://www.herbs.org

National Center for Complementary and Alternative Medicine (NCCAM)
National Institutes of Health
NCCAM Clearinghouse
P.O. Box 7923
Gaithersburg, MD 20898
tel: 888.644.6266 ❧ fax: 866.464.3616
http://nccam.nih.gov

National Center for Homeopathy (NCN)
801 North Fairfax St. Ste. 306
Alexandria, VA 22314
tel: 703.548.7790 ❧ fax: 703.548.7792
www.homeopathic.org

National Choice Directory
4957 Lakemont Blvd SE, Ste. C4-20
Bellevue, WA 98006
tel: 425.375.1987 or 800.465.0595
fax: 425.988.0160
www.naturalchoice.com

National Council for Reliable Health Information
300 East Pink Hill Rd.
Independence, MO 64057
tel: 816.228.4595
http://ncahf.org

National Institutes of Health
Office of Dietary Supplements
Building 21, Room 1825
31 Center Dr., MSC 2086
Bethesda, MD 20892
tel: 301.435.2920 ❧ fax: 301.480.1945
http://www.nlm.nih.gov

Sage Mountain Herbal Retreat Center and Botanical Sanctuary
Sage
P.O.Box 420
E. Barre, VT 05649
tel: 802.479.9825 ❧ fax: 802.476.3722
http://www.sagemountain.com

The US Department of Health and Human Services
200 Independence Ave. S.W.
Washington, DC 20201
tel: 202.619.0257 ❧ fax: 877.696.6775
http://www.hhs.gov

United Plant Savers
P.O. Box 400
East Barre, VT 05649
tel: 802.467.6487 ❧ fax: 802.476.3722
http://www.unitedplantsavers.com

U.S. Food and Drug Administration
Center for Food Safety and Applied Nutrition
5600 Fishers Lane
Rockville, MD 20857
Toll free information line:
888.463.6332
http://www.fda.gov

Women to Women Personal Program
Helping a million women a year with a natural approach to health.
P.O. Box 306
Portland, ME 04112
tel: 800.207.8193 (the Personal Program)
tel: 800.340.5382 (the Healthcare Center)
http://womentowomen.com

Natural Products Association (NNFA),
Promoting products for healthy lifestyles
1773 T St. NW
Washington, DC 20009
tel: 202.223.0101 ❧ fax: 202.223.0250
— and —
2112 E Fourth St. Ste. 200
Santa Ana, CA 92705
tel: 714.460.7732 or 800.966.6632
fax: 714.460.7444
www.nnfa.org

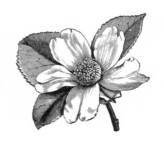

Glossary

ALKALOID: a naturally occurring amine (organic compound) produced by a plant.

CLEANSING ALTERNATIVE: a cleansing using natural products and methods.

AMBER: a fossil resin, a gemstone.

ANALGESIC: a remedy that relieves pain, colloquially known as a painkiller.

ANAPHYLAXIS: a severe and rapid multi-system allergic reaction.

ANTIBIOTIC: destroys or inhibits the growth of microorganisms.

ANTIMICROBIAL: destroys microorganisms.

ANTIOXIDANTS: ingredients used as dietary supplements for healthy purposes to prevent cancer or heart disease by reducing oxidation.

ANTISEPTIC: prevents the growth and reproduction of bacteria, fungi, viruses on the external surface of the body.

ANXIETY: a complex combination of emotions that includes fear and worry.

AMPELOTHERAPY: a system of natural rejuvenating treatment with grapes.

ASTRIGENT: precipitates proteins from the surface of cells or mucous membranes.

BACTERICIDAL: disinfectants killing bacteria.

BOREDOM: a state of mind in which one interprets the environment as dull and not stimulating.

CONCOCTION: to prepare or make by combining ingredients, usually medicinal herbs.

DECOCTION: an extract of the essence of herbs obtained by simmering the herbs in water for 30 minutes to one hour until the volume has been recduced by one-third.

DECOMPOSITION: biological process through which organic material is reduced.

DIGESTION: the process of metabolism whereby a biological entity processes a substance in order to convert the substance into nutrients.

DISTRESS: stress caused by adverse events; acute physical or mental suffering.

DIURETIC: a medicine or substance that increases urine flow.

ESSENTIAL OIL: volatile oil extracted from plants, containing a mixture of active constituents, highly aromatic.

EXPECTORANT: encourages the removal of phlegm from the respiratory tract.

FASTING: the act of willingly abstaining from some or all food including some drinks, for a period of time.

FATIGUE: weariness from bodily or mental exertion. Chronic fatigue syndrome—a central nervous system disease.

FEBRIFUGE: reduces fever.

GRECHIKHA: the Russian word for buckwheat.

HAPPINESS: an emotional or affective state that feels good or pleasing.

HOMESICKNESS: a feeling of longing for familiar surroundings.

HYPERTENSION: high blood pressure.

HYPOTENSION: low blood pressure.

IMMUNE SYSTEM: protects the body from infection.

INFLAMMATION: the first response of the immune system to infection or irritation.

INFUSION: a method of preparing a natural medicinal drink in which 1-2 teaspoons of dried herbs or 1-4 teaspoons of fresh flowers or berries are placed in boiling water to steep for 7-10 minutes.

INTESTINE: the lower part of the alimentary canal extending from the stomach to the anus.

KASHA: a porridge made with wheat, rice, buckwheat, oats, millet. One of the oldest meals in Eastern European cuisine, "the original mother of bread."

KISSEL: the Russian word for a kind of starchy jelly.

MEDITATION: a variety of contempletive practices with different goals for personal development, to achieve eternal peace and to be healthier.

METABOLISM: the biochemical modification of chemical compounds in living organisms and cells.

NASTOYKA: the russian word for a specially prepared liquor or infusion.

NEPHRITIS: inflammation of the kidney.

OTITIS: a general term for inflammation or infection of the ear.

OXYGEN: the second most common element on Earth.

PHLEGM: the sticky liquid secreted by the mucous membranes.

PHYTONCIDES: antimicrobial allelochemic volatile organic compounds derived from plants.

PHYSICAL THERAPY (PHYSIOTHERAPY): a system of prevention, promotion, treatment and rehabilitation, helping people to develop, maintain and restore maximum movement and functional ability throughout the lifespan.

PHYTOTHERAPY (HERBALISM, HERBAL MEDICINE): a folk and traditional medicinal practice based on the use of plants and plant extracts.

PREVENTION: any activity that avoids the development of a disease.

PREVENTIVE MEDICINE: a part of medicine engaged with preventing disease rather than curing it.

REGENERATION: the ability to recreate lost or damaged tissues, organs and limbs.

REJUVENATION: to restore to youthful vigor.

RESPIRATORY: a system of humans and other mammals comprising the lungs and other organs involved in breathing.

SENSITIVITY: rapid perception with the senses, reacting to small changes, degree of susceptibility to stimulation.

STRESS: the sum of physical and mental responses to an unacceptable imparity between real or imagined personal experience and personal expectations.

TANNINS: astringent, bitter-tasting plant polyphenols (a group of chemical substances found in plants) that bind and precipitate proteins.

TINCTURE: a solution made by steeping the dried or fresh herbs in a mixture of alcohol and water.

TONIC: nourishing, restoring, and supporting for the whole body.

TOXIN: a poisonous substance produced by living cells or organisms.

YOGA: means *Union* in Sanskrit, a system of ancient spiritual practices that originated in India and remains a vibrant tradition as the means of enlightenment of life.

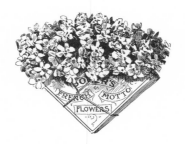

Bibliography

Apollodorus, *Mythology Library*, Leningrad: Science, 1972

(Apollodorus *Bibliotheca* (Library of Greek Mythology), today often called Pseudo-Apollodorus)

Ashukin, N., Ashukin, M., *Aphorisms, Quotations, Sayings,* Moscow: Goslitizdat, 1955.

Akchurin, R., *Secrets of a Sunny Berry: Proverbs, Sayings, Legends,* Kishinev: 1965.

Blair, Nancy, *The Book of Goddesses,* London: Vega, 2002

Bown, Deni, *The Herb Society of America: Encyclopedia of Herbs and Their Uses.* New York: Dorling Kindersley Publishing, 1995.

Brief Medical Encyclopedia, V.1-3, Moscow: Prosveschthenie, 1972.

Coates, P., Blackman, M., Cragg, G., et al, eds. *Encyclopedia of Dietary Supplements,* New York, NY: Marcel Dekker, 2005.

Dioscorides, *De Materia Medica,* trans. John Godyer 1655, ed. R.T. Gunther 1933, Oxford University Press (1934).

Encyclopedia of People's Medicine, Moscow: ANS, 1994; Moscow: Ekoizdat, Publishing House Konstantin Klimenko, 1993.

English-Russian Medical Dictionary, 2nd Edition, stereotyped. Moscow: Russky Yazyk Publishers, 1992.

English-Russian Dictionary of Chemistry and Chemical Technology, Second stereotype edition. ed. V.V. Kafarov, Academician, "Russo", Moscow, 1995; "Technica Ltd.", Moscow, 1995.

English-Russian Dictionary of Food Industry, 3rd stereotype edition. ed. L.P. Kovalskaya, Dr. of Science "Russo", Moscow 1995.

Fetrow, Charles, W. Pharm. D., Avila Juan, R. Pharm. D. *The Complete Guide to Herbal Medicines*. New York, London, Toronto, Sydney, Singapore: Pocket Books, a division of Simon & Schuster, Inc., 2000.

Gerard, John, *The Herball or General Historie of Plantes,* 1597. First modern edition by Marcus Woodward 1927 published 1931. Leaves from Gerard's Herball arranged for Garden Lovers by Marcus Woodward with 130 illustrations after the original woodcuts. Printed in the British Isles: Gerald Howe Ltd., 1931.

Grieve, Maud, *A Modern Herbal,* New York: Harcourt, Brace & Co., 1931. Reprint edition. New York: Dover Publications, 1971.

Griggs, Barbara, *Green Pharmacy.* New York: Viking, 1982. Reprint edition, Rochester, Vermont: Healing Arts Press, 1991.

Hoffman, David. *The Herbal Handbook, a User's Guide to Medicinal Herbalism.* Rochester, Vermont: Healing Arts Press, 1987.

Hiller, Malcolm, *The Little Scented Library: Wreaths and Garlands.* London, Great Britain by Dorling Kindersley Limited, New York: Simon and Schuster, 1992.

J.M.Nickell's, *Botanical Ready Reference.* Especially designed for Druggists and Physicians. Containing all of the botanical drugs, known up to the present time, giving their medicinal properties, and all of their Botanical, Common, Pharmacopoeial and German Common (in German) names. With an introduction to this special edition by Herb Sed. First reprint by M.L.Baker, 1972. New material 1976 by Trinity Center Press; Banning, California: Enos Publishing Co.1976.

Kloss, Jethro. *Back to Eden.* A Human Interest Story of Health and Restoration to be Found in Herb, Root, and Bark. Revised and expanded second edition. Kloss Family Heirloom edition. Loma Linda, California: Back to Eden Books Publishing Vo., An Enterprise of The Jethro Kloss Family, 1994.

Krieger, Anna, *The Pocket Guide to Herbs,* London, Great Britain: Parkgate Books, Ltd., 1992

Kun, N.A., Neickhardt, A.A., *Legends of Ancient Greece and Ancient Rome,* Moscow: Pravda Publishers, 1987

Lavabre, Marcel, *Aromatherapy Workbook.* Rochester, Vermont: Healing Arts Press, 1990.

Hudges, Holly, Compiled, *Meditations On The Earth.* A Celebration of Nature in Quotations, Poems and Essays, Philadelphia-London: Running Press 1994.

Muir, John, *The Mountains of California,* New York: The Century Co. 1894

Murray, Michael, *The Healing Power of Herbs.* Rocklin, California: Prima Publishing, 1992

Murray, Michael, N.D. *The Pill Book to Natural Medicines.* New York, Toronto, London, Sydney, Auckland: Batnam Books, 2002

Ody, Penelope, *The Complete Medicinal Herbal.* New York: Dorling Kindersley Inc., 1993

Pliny *Natural History* tran. W.H.S. Jones, 10 volumes. Cambridge: Harvard University Press, 1956.

Pushkin, Alexander, Poem "Ruslan and Ludmila," trans. and retold S. Konnikova, 3 volumes, volume 1, Moscow: Artistic Literature, 1985.

Randckhava, M., *Gardens Through the Centuries.* Moscow: Knowledge, 1999.

Seaman, Barbara, *The Doctor's Case Against Pill.* New York: Avon Books, a Division of the Hearst Corporation, 1970.

Sokolov Sergey, Zamotaev Ivan, *Guide to Medicinal Plants* (Phytotherapy), Moscow: Medicine, 1984.

The New College Latin & English Dictionary. Revised and Enlarged by John C. Traupman, Ph.D., St.Joseph's University, Philadelphia. New York, Toronto, London, Sydney, Auckland, Batnam Books, 1966

Thoreau, Henri David, *A Week on the Concord and Merrimack Rivers,* 1849, first book written during his stay at Walden Pond.

Tyler, V.E. *The Honest Herbal,* 3rd edition. Binghamton, NY: Pharmaceutical Products Press, 1993.

Vogel, H.C.A., *The Nature Doctor. A Manuel of Traditional and Complementary Medicine.* New Canaan, Connecticut: Keats Publishing, 1991.

Vescolli, Michael, *The Celtic Tree Calendar. Your Tree Sign and You,* London: Souvenir Press and Rosemary Dear, 1999, p. 6

Verzilin, Nikolai, *Follow Robinson,* Leningrad: Children's Literature, 1974, p.163

Wigmore, Ann, *Be Your Own Doctor. How to Use Nature as a Healer and Builder of Health.* A Positive Guide to Natural Living. Wayne, New Jersey: Avery Publishing Group, 1982.

Zakharov, V., Djungietu, E., *Health is in Our Hands.* A Compilation of Proverbs, Sayings and Aphorisms, Kishinev: Shteentsa, 1972.

Zamiatina, Natalia, *Medicinal Plants,* Moscow: ABF, 1998.

Zolotnitsky, N.F., *Flowers in Legends and Tales.* St. Petersburg, Russia, ed. A.F. Devrien, 1911.

All folk tales, fairy tales, myths, stories and ancient legends included in this book have been adapted by the author from her family's foretelling, diaries and notes. The following tales have been translated and retold by Svetlana Konnikova:

A Little Story about My Grandpa and His Grapevine of Happiness
Ampelos, a Remarkable Daughter
How a Boy "Ampel" Became a Magnificent Grape Star
How Brave Storks Saved Soldiers from Death
Twelve Months
One Hundred Brains
Green Savior
How God Created 70 Medicinal Herbs
Masha, a Little Scarlet Flower and the Beast
Chamomile, a Passenger without a Ticket
On the Ruins of Jurate's Amber Castle
A Sunny Stone with a Silver Snake Inside
The Tale of the Firebird, Tsarevich Ivan and the Gray Wolf
How Goddess Flora Created a Name for One Tiny Flower
Pan and Syringe
Lilacs, the Flowers Sprinkled by the Spring
How a Magical Elixir of Life Put Nature to Sleep
Valley of Flowers (Tofalgarski folklore, oral tradition)
Andersen, Hans Christian, Public Domain, English translation: H.P. Paul (1872) used for educational and informational purposes:
The Elf of the Rose, 1839
Under the Willow Tree, 1853
The Little Elder Tree, 1872
The Buckwheat, 1842
The Snowdrop, 1863
Little Ida's Flowers, 1835
The Candles, 1870

Publications and Periodicals

Cheraskin, E., MD., DMD., Journal of Orthomolecular Medicine, 9:1, first quarter 1994, p.39-45

Journal of Allergy and Clinical Immunology, 103:559 -62, 1999

Chinese Herbal Remedies in Childhood Eczema, The Lancet, March 31, 1990, 795

Health, United States, 2002 with Chartbook on Trends in the Health of Americans, National Center for Health Statistics Report, September 12, 2002

Center for Disease Control National Center for Health Statistics, May 27, 2004 (20-page full text PDF report).

National Institutes of Health, National Health, Lung and Blood Institute. Data release for World Asthma Day, May 2001.

National Ambulatory Medical Care Survey: 2001 Summary

National Hospital Ambulatory Medical Care Survey: 2002 Emergency Department Summary.

Natural Medicines Comprehensive Database Web site.

President's Task Force on Environmental Health Risks and Safety to Children. Asthma and the Environment: A Strategy to Protect Children. Revised May 2000.

Research on essential foundation: Chapter 14—Outdoor Recreation in America's Parks and Recreation, August 2002; http:uuufindarticles.com

The Teachings of Integral Yoga by Sri Swani Satchidananda, www.yogaville.org

U.S. Department of Health and Human Services. "Tracking Healthy People 2010." Section 24—Respiratory Diseases, November 2000. The national data system I, the National Hospital Discharge Survey conducted by the National Center for Health Statistics. http://www.cgc.gov

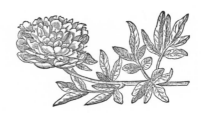

Useful Addresses / Herbal Suppliers

You can buy and learn more about herbs, nutritional supplements and natural foods by contacting the companies and organizations below. Many of them have Web addresses. Keep in mind that these addresses may change without notice. Inclusion in the following list doesn't indicate endorsement of any company or organization by the author or publisher.

Avena Botanicals, 219 Mill St.
Rockport, ME 04856
tel: 207.594.0694 ❧ fax: 866.282.8362
http://www.avenaherbs.com

Blessed Herbs, 109 Bare Plains Road
Oakham, MA 01068
tel: 1-800-489-HERB (4372)
fax: 508-882-3755
http://www.blessedherbs.com

Blessed Maine Herb Farm, 257
Chapman Ridge
Athens, ME 04912
tel: 207.654.2879
http://www.blessedmaineherbs.com

Classic Soap Shoppe, 1804 Hwy 206
Cisco, TX 76437
tel: 254.442.2630
http://www.classicsoapshoppe.com

Diamond Organics, 1272 Highway 1
Moss Landing, CA 95039
tel: 888.674.2642 ❧ fax: 888.888.6777
http://www.diamondorganics.com

Herb Pharm
202260 Williams Hwy
Williams, OR 97544
tel: 541.846.6262 ❧ fax: 800.545.7392
http://www.herb-pharm.com

Mayway Corporation
1338 Mandela Street,
Oakland, CA 94607
tel: 800-262-9929 or 510-208-3113
fax: 800-909-2828 or 510-208-3069
http://www.mayway.com

Frontier Natural Products Co-op
P.O. Box 299, 3021 78th St.
Norway, IA 52318
tel: 800-669-3275 ❧ fax: 800-717-4372
http://www.frontiercoop.com

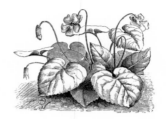

Index

A

abrasions, 30.
  See also wound remedies
acetylsalicylic acid (aspirin), 77
acne remedies, 9, 30, 99
Adam, Eve, and the snowdrops,
  195
Adams, Richard, 175
adaptation, human ability
  for, 25
Addison, Joseph, 84, 126
Aeschylus, 150
Aesculapius/Asclepiad, 28–29
agrimony, 101, 102
air pollution, 108–9, 211, 216,
  236
alcohol intake, 141
alimentary canal problems,
  37, 141
allergens, 88, 111–12, 193
allergic contact dermatitis, 92
allergic rhinitis, 85, 86, 90–91,
  103–4.
  See also sinus problems
allergies: about, 85–87, 93;
  ailments from, 90–91;
  author's experience with, 93–
  95; irritants, 88–89; physical
  factors, 90; prevention of, 87,
  95–98; symptoms of, 91–93
allergy remedies for adults,
  99–107
allergy remedies for children,
  113–20
almond oil, 192, 193

almonds, for cleansing, 18,
  38, 87
aloe vera, 12–13, 220, 245
alternative medicine, 7–8, 11,
  16–17, 28
Alzheimer's disease, 177
amber: about, 146–48, 254;
  folk tales about, 131–32,
  148–49; healing properties
  of, 127–30, 146, 148
American Council for
  Headache Education, 132–33
American Heart Association, 39
American Lung Association,
  85–86
ammonia or ammonia capsule,
  215, 216
ampelotherapy, 42–45
anaphylaxis, incidence of, 86
Andersen, Hans Christian: on
  buckwheat, 182–83; elder
  tree mother story, 159; "Little
  Ida's Flowers," 198, 199; on
  living, 3; reading stories by,
  225; "The Candles," 225–26;
  "The Elf of the Rose," 74–75;
  "The Snowdrop," 194, 195;
  "Under the Willow Tree,"
  77, 78
anemia, headaches related to,
  138–39
anemia, remedies for: beets,
  17, 18; lemon balm,
  144–45; nettle mixture, 102;
  sweetbrier/rose hips, 64

animal instincts, 8–9, 10,
  19–20
animals: as irritants, 88, 103–4,
  112, 120–22; as pets, 199
anise and anise seeds: for
  asthma, 218, 220; for colds,
  77; essential oil from, 223;
  as stimulating aroma, 193
antibacterials: garlic, 30, 220;
  geranium, 216; grapes,
  44–45; lysozyme, 11; Mary's
  Root powder, 103; onion,
  71; potato juice, 33; saunas,
  238; sphagnum moss, 15;
  trees, 61, 108–9, 238.
  See also essential oils
antibiotics, 11–13, 23, 73,
  86, 93
antifungals, 30, 92
anti-inflammatories: beets,
  19; birch, 58; buckthorn
  and black elder, 74;
  calendula, 145; color red,
  106–7; Greater celandine,
  103; honey, 34; linden,
  79; lungwort, 82; marsh
  cudweed, 59, 66; pine bath,
  166, 236; potato poultice,
  34; potato starch, 35; St.
  John's Wort, 142; white oak,
  61; white willow, 77
antioxidants, 39–40
antiseptics: citrus fruits, 81;
  elder flowers, 79; garlic, 9,
  30; grape juice, 37;

cleansing herbs and plants (cont.)
Cleansing Maid, 87; fennel, 59, 60; geraniums, 216; Greater celandine, 103; green tea, 95, 96; herbal teas, 97–98; horsetail, 87; licorice root, 59, 60; nettle, 61, 97; peppermint, 56, 57, 76, 87; rose hips, 96; sage, 76; strawberries, 98; wild marjoram, 56–57; willow bark, 58, 77. *See also* cleansing foods
cleansing methods: about, 87; for allergy prevention, 87, 95–99; diaphoretics, 56, 57, 58, 70; diuretics, 19, 76, 99, 103, 219; enemas, 70, 135, 139, 176; fasting, 55, 56, 70; infusions, 56–61; need for, 53, 87, 133, 238; restoration remedies, 98; rules for, 55; showers three times a day, 105; sleep, 55, 98; tinctures, 76; vitamin teas, 96–97. *See also* baths; expectorants; herbal baths
clover, for headaches, 144
coffee, 30, 101, 138, 155
cognac, 170
Cold Punch recipe, 170
colds: about, 53; from allergic reactions, 89; as body's cleansing process, 55–56; in children, 115–16; complications from, 72; headaches related to, 145–46; sore throat, 33, 68–69, 81, 89. *See also* congestion remedies; flu
cold remedies, **56–61, 64–69**; beets, 18; cyclamen, 245; elecampane, 143; herbal baths, 60–61; oat straw, 83; onion drops, 63; potato "tea," 33
cold remedies for children, **115–16**
cold water self-cure technique, 155

colewort, 99
colors for healing, 106–7, 160–61
coltsfoot, 56–57, 77, 130, 216
communication skills, 263, 265–68
Complete Guide to Herbal Medicines (Fetrow and Avila), 38–39
Complete Medicinal Herbal (Ody), 91
compresses, oak bark, 61
congestion, 88, 89, 91
congestion remedies: aloe vera, 12; beets, 18; black elder, 79, 82; elecampane, 143; honey, 29, 55, 57, 58, 59, 81; massage, 64; nettle mixture, 102; potatoes, 31, 82, 216; remedy, 57; tree besoms, 238. *See also* inhalation therapy
coniferous trees and bushes, 210, 214
conjunctivitis, 89, **103–4,** 113
constipation, 18, 176. *See also* laxatives
contrast baths, 136
conventional medicine. *See* traditional medicine
corn silk, for dermatitis, 100
corns, remedies for, 9, 30, 34
cotton fabric for children, 113
coughs, 29, 59, 72, 88, 143. *See also* bronchial asthma; bronchitis; colds; congestion remedies
Cousteau, Jacques Yves, 150
cranberries: for cleansing, 97; for dermatitis, 100; for headaches, 136; in vitamin teas, 169, 239
crane and fox fable, 62–63
Crimean vacations, 214, 230–35
Curie, Marie, 110
cyclamen flowers, 245
cypress trees: as author's talisman, 230–35; as relaxing aroma, 193; in "Three Daughters, Three Trees," 242–43

D

daisies, for bruises and sprains, 10
dandelion root: for allergic reactions, 100, 103, 115, 116; for metabolism, 116
Da Vinci, Leonardo, 50, 173
dental health, 43
depression, remedies for, 37, 38, 141, 142. *See also* nervous disorders
dermatitis, sources of, 88, 91–93
dermatitis remedies, **99–100, 105–6, 115–16**; aloe, 12; birch vodka or tincture, 58; Black Knight nastoyka, 105; cabbage, 99; elecampane, 143; garlic clove juice, 30; grape leaf preparations, 48; jojoba oil, 192; lily bulb with honey, 212; oak bark, 61; potato poultice, 34. *See also* eczema
dermatitis remedies for children, 115–16
diaphoretics: for colds, 56–57, 58, 79; for flu, 70, 73, 79
diathesis, 112, 113–14, 120
digestive system: diet for, 177; and fatigue, 176; and food allergies, 89; intestinal support, 18–19, 47, 107
digestive system remedies, **139–40, 177–78**; beets, 18; black tea, 47; burdock root, 115; cyclamen, 245; dill, 165; milk, 69; nettle mixture, 102; potato juice, 32, 33; rose hips, 65; valerian root, 141; wood betony, 76
dill, 160, 165, 168
discoid eczema, 92
disinfectants: herbal bath as, 120; medicinal plants, 222; mint as internal, 176; pine oil, 236, 238; in sphagnum moss, 15; thyme, 222
distress vs. good stress, 189–90, 193–94. *See also* managing stress; stress as distress

linden (cont.)
  for tension or headaches,
    137, 191
listening, 5, 189
Lithuania, "the land of amber,"
  127–30
"Little Ida's Flowers"
  (Andersen), 198, 199
liver health support: beets, 18,
  19; birch vodka or tincture,
  58; color purple, 107; garden
  radish juice, 29; grapes, 37;
  Greater celandine, 103; wood
  betony, 76
lotus aroma, 222
lungs, warning about grape
  therapy and, 43.
  See also congestion remedies
lungwort, 82
lymph system, 39
lysozyme, 11

M

magnesium, 190
Mama's memos about children,
  265–68
Mama's Onion Salad recipe, 98
managing stress: aromatherapy,
  192–93; exercise, 193;
  hydrotherapy, 191–93;
  intellectual stimulation, 200–
  201; pets for, 199; proper
  nutrition, 190–91
maple trees, 246, 247, 249
marsh cudweed, 59, 66–67
marshmallow, for colds, 56–57,
  60
Mary's Root powder, 103
"Mashed Onions," 220
massage: for asthmatic attacks,
  215; for blood circulation,
  39, 156, 191–92; with dry-
  skin brush, 191–92; for
  headaches, 64, 136, 138; for
  insomnia, 156; self-massage,
  191
Materia Medica (Theophrastus),
  275–76
McPhee, John, 109
measles, buckwheat for, 179
medical mistakes, 26–27

Medicinal Matters
  (Theophrastus), 275–76
medicinal plants, steaming,
  221–22
menopausal symptom remedies,
  130, 142, 165
menthol, 60
Mercola, Joseph, 27
metabolism support: and
  allergy-related problems in
  children, 115–16; beets, 18;
  farmer's cheese, 95; grapes,
  37; herbal rejuvenating bath,
  120; hops-filled pillow, 213;
  Mama's Onion Salad, 98
migraine headaches: about,
  132–34; chemicals for, 29;
  remedies for, 136, 142, 165
milk: for cleansing, 68; for
  energy, 186, 210; for
  insomnia, 157; as natural
  healer, 69; for respiratory
  problems, 71, 81; for sound
  sleep, 178; sweet sauce for
  kasha, 180
Milk Punch recipe, 170
milk scabs on children, 112
Milne, A. A., 259
mineral water, 43, 68, 190, 217
mint: in calming tea, 168; in
  diaphoretic infusion, 58; for
  dizziness, 176–77; essential
  oil from, 223; for flu, 70;
  for insomnia, 168; for
  nervous system, 210. See also
  peppermint
mistletoe berries, warning
  about, 164
mistletoe, for insomnia, 164
mold, 11, 12–13, 111–12
Moldova, Russia: childhood
  memories, 22–23;
  description of, 50; Herculean
  oak in, 249–53; white storks
  in, 45–46; winter memories,
  223–25
Monet, Claude, 201
Montaigne, Michel Euquem
  de, 110
morphine poisoning, grapes

for, 37
Moscow State University, stories
  from, 160–61, 186–89,
  193–94
moss, 14–15
Mother Nature: body cleansing
  process and, 55; communing
  with, 209; gifts from, 10;
  harmony with, 9; healing
  power of, 178; humanity's
  separation from, 211;
  learning about, 240–41;
  mother archetype, 261,
  265–68; as talented artist,
  248–49
motherwort, 105, 163, 164,
  169
motivation, philosophy for, 5–6
mountain ash berries, for
  cleansing, 97
Mountain Cranberry tree, 243
mucous membranes: and
  allergic reactions, 91, 112;
  and bronchial asthma, 214;
  and Flonase, 95; flu or colds
  and, 72; remedies for, 82,
  103–4, 113–14, 116, 217;
  sensitivity of, 112, 133; wine
  with baking soda for, 216
Muir, John, 109, 246–47, 260
mulberry trees, 245
mullein, 58, 66, 82
Muscat grapes, 44
music for relaxing, 193
mustard plaster for asthmatic
  attack, 215

N

nail biting, aloe for, 12
nastoykas: about, 102, 130,
  141, 205–6; for allergic
  conditions, 102, 104; for
  bronchial asthma, 221; for
  insomnia, 141–42, 163; for
  nervous disorders, 163; for
  skin problems, 48, 105
National Center for Health
  Statistics (NCHS), 53
National Institute of Allergy
  and Infectious Diseases
  (NIAID), 85–86

V

valerian: about, 142; for allergic reactions, 105; in calming tea, 168, 169; essential oil from, 223; for headaches, 141; for insomnia, 163, 164, 165, 166, 168; for insomnia or nervousness, 141–42, 157; for relaxing bath, 166
"Valley of Flowers," 268, 269–72
vanilla extract, 81, 170
vapors. *See* inhalation therapy
varicose eczema, 92
vascular health support: beets, 18; citrus fruits, 80; gooseberries, 105; grapes, 45; milk, 69; rose hips tea, 59. *See also* blood circulation
vegetable puree for infants, 114
vegetables: for breaking a fast, 70; for cleansing, 98; as "food therapy," 144; Latin names for, 276–81. *See also specific vegetables*
vegetative neurosis, violet for, 107
verbena, 245
Verzilin, Nikolai, 14
Vindemiatrix (grape star), 41–42
vinegar: for asthmatic attack, 215; for bathing, 73, 223; compress, for headache, 135; for rheumatism, 38. *See also* apple cider vinegar
viral infections, 61
Vitachella, 22–23

vitamin B complex, 73, 137
vitamin C for flu or colds, 72, 73, 137
vitamin P, 179
vitamin teas, 96–97, 169, 238–39
Vitis-Isabella grapes, 44
vodka, 102, 115, 168, 176. *See also* nastoykas
Vogel, H. C. A., 88
Vostokov, Victor F., 245

W

walnuts: for cleansing, 177; for fatigue and headaches, 210; for immune system, 47; for nervous system, 38; in Red Wheels salads, 19; in Vitachella, 22–23
warts, apples for, 30
weight loss, 30, 107
wheat bran for rejuvenating bath, 119, 120
white oak bark, 61
white willow bark, 77
white wine. *See* wine
Wigmore, Ann, 178
wild lettuce/garden lettuce, 66, 162
wild marjoram: for allergic reactions, 119; for asthma, 218, 220; for colds/cleansing, 56–57; for insomnia, 164, 165; for rejuvenating bath, 119, 120; for sore throat, 68–69; in vitamin teas, 239
willow bark, 58, 59, 77, 219
wine: antioxidants in, 40; with

dill, for sleep, 160, 168; from elderberries, 82; in herbal bath, 73; for insomnia, 160; for longevity and vitality, 141; for mucus dilution, 216; in punch recipes, 170; for respiratory disorders, 220; for Sweet Kiss recovery drink, 68
winter in Moldova, Russia, 223–25
Wolfe, Thomas, 84
women: stress levels of, 185; working away from home, 262–64
wood betony, for flu, 76
Wooden Leg, 260
Wordsworth, William, 202
working women, stress levels of, 185
World Health Organization, 27
wound remedies: agrimony bath, 101; aloe, 12; cabbage juice, 99; calendula, 145; moss, 14–15; St. John's Wort, 142; yarrow leaves, 10

Y

Yalta, discovery of, 232–33
yarrow: in calming tea, 168; for eczema, 101; for insomnia, 168; for metabolism, 116; for rejuvenating bath, 119; for wounds and nosebleed, 10
yeast growth, 92
yellow melilot, for insomnia, 164

Z

Zyrtec, 94–95

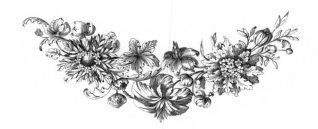

Credits

Michael Vescolli, *The Celtic Tree Calendar. Your Tree Sign and You.* Translated from German by Rosemary Dear. London: Souvenir Press, Ltd. Copyright © 1999 by Souvenir Press and Rosemary Dear. The Celtic Tree Calendar, p.6 reprinted by permission of the publisher.

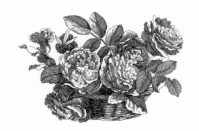

Acknowledgments

I extend my heartfelt thanks to those who have contributed to this book. I greatly appreciate the expertise, advice and encouragement from my favorite doctors, Anna Maria Clement and Brian Clement, codirectors of Hippocrates Health Institute (West Palm Beach, Florida).

Many thanks to Jan Marie Werblin Kemp who laid the groundwork for this book, supported me with all my ideas, and taught me that if you have a dream, go for it.

Loving thanks to Judy King, for helping refine my manuscript, for her integrity, and sense of quality and loyalty which is truly rare to find today.

Special thanks to my illustrator Anatoli Smishliaev. Your encouragement, beloved friendship and creativity are greatly appreciated.

I feel a deep sense of gratitude for the creation of this book to:

- all the wise, insightful women in my family;

- the happy memory of my grandma, grandpa, and my wonderful, erudite father;

- my wise, protective Mama Lubov (her name means "love" in English) for her expertise, support, devotion, and constant love. Her presence in my life is invaluable;

- my husband, Greg; and my sons, Vitaly and Yuri, who encouraged me to go for my dreams and are the dearest and most treasured people in my life.

I love all of you—you are the best.

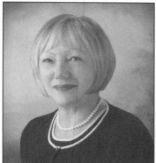

A Note About the Author

SVETLANA KONNIKOVA grew up in Moldova (located between Romania and Ukraine) amidst medical professionals active in natural medicine, folk healers and herbalists, grape growers and winemakers. Svetlana holds a master's degree in journalism from Moscow State University and an associate's degree in nursing. While living in the former Soviet Union she wrote nonfiction books, many award-winning television scripts and hosted several television shows, including Listen and Learn, Masterpieces of World Literature and Science and Life. She is a member of the American Botanical Council and an avid researcher of herbal medicines, healthy lifestyles and holistic health practices that combine contemporary thought with the world's great spiritual, cultural and healing traditions.

www.aurorapublishers.com   www.mamashomeremedies.com

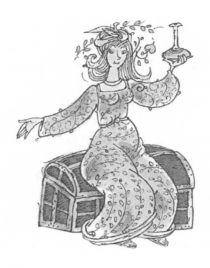

I didn't get here by dreaming about it or thinking about it
– I got here by doing it.

— Estée Lauder, cosmetics company founder

Editors: Jan Marie Werblin Kemp, Judy King

Cover design by Janice M. Phelps

Book design by Peri Poloni-Gabriel, www.knockoutbooks.com

Layout design by Monica Thomas

Index by Melody Englund

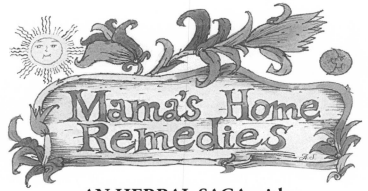

AN HERBAL SAGA with
TIME-TESTED SECRETS of GOOD HEALTH
and NATURAL LIVING, HIDDEN UNTIL NOW
"UNDER SEVEN SEALS"

Vividly descriptive, helpful and nurturing, this ultimate natural home remedies book arrives just in time to help you change the way you live and think about life's dilemma—how to improve and maintain your health and happiness for many years to come. Colorfully written with all-inclusive artist's palette, *Mama's Home Remedies* presents to the reader a spectacular kaleidoscopic tapestry woven of centuries-old herbal remedies, timeless techniques and concepts, intellectual rigor and joyfully recounted anecdotes and folk tales, women's wisdom, family values and traditions, artistically rendered illustrations and an abundance of humor—all that we hold sacred in life.

Many years ago Mama would gather "the girls" (medical professionals like she was) for tea each Friday in her fragrant, blossoming garden in Moldova. Under a canopy of trees filled with birdsong they'd strengthen their bond of friendship and share stories of the success they'd achieved using natural remedies to treat and heal their patients and neighbors. As each woman recounted her experiences, Mama's daughter, 12-year-old Svetlana, sat attentively on a bench recording in her journal "recipes" for teas, tinctures, infusions and poultices.

Mama's Home Remedies is a collection of the abundant knowledge of natural health and healing that the young Svetlana garnered in Mama's tea garden, intertwined with her grandmother's fairy tales, family vignettes, legends and herbal lore. Filled with easy-to-make, natural, healing recipes for common ailments and illnesses—such as allergies, headaches, stress, fatigue, insomnia, asthma, and respiratory problems—this all-encompassing guide to wellness offers a holistic approach that blends alternative treatments with folklore, psychology, philosophy, and spirituality to foster optimal health and joyful living.